TITANIC

Paul Brooke

MINERVA PRESS
MONTREUX   LONDON   WASHINGTON

TITANIC
Copyright © Paul Brooke 1995

All Rights Reserved

ISBN 1 85863 412 1

First published 1995 by
MINERVA PRESS
1 Cromwell Place
London SW7 2JE

Printed in Great Britain
Antony Rowe Ltd., Chippenham, Wiltshire.

TITANIC

I dedicate this book to Joanne, my long suffering love, without whose help it might never have been written, and to Lennie, Vi, Denis and Freda, Harry and Donna, without whose faith it might never have been published: also to Tyler Brooke, my first grandson, and future inspiration. Thank you all, from the bottom of my heart.

About the Author

Paul Brooke was born in Northern Rhodesia (Zambia) in 1942, and came to England, aged thirteen, when his father retired from the Colonial Service, having been educated in East London, South Africa and Purley, Surrey.

He has combined a successful career in the Leisure Industry with a life-long interest in his homeland, and is currently engaged in writing a quinary, set in Southern Africa, amongst other projects. He is married, and lives overlooking the sea in Sussex, another of his keen interests.

FOREWORD

On 1st September 1985, Dr Robert Ballard, of the Woods Hole Oceanographic Institute, found the last resting place of RMS *Titanic*, after an extensive search, off the coast of Newfoundland: but not in her last reported position. She was 12,500 feet down, in complete darkness, broken in two by her ordeal, but still remarkably well preserved after seventy-three years. The only way to reach her - at that great depth - was by mini-submarine, especially designed to withstand the enormous pressure; and equipped to photograph and collect debris which fell out of the illustrious ship when she sank. The mini-sub *Alvin* was used to map the wreck-site and, during a later Franco-American expedition, the *Nautile* completed the task.

It was hoped the discovery would answer many questions as to how the "unsinkable" liner was lost. While it achieved this, to some extent, it raised a new set of queries over what actually happened on the fateful night; 14-15th April 1912. The evidence of the camera casts doubt on the whole story as glibly delivered to the world; on the honesty of the ship's owners; on the motives of the crew; on the integrity of some of the passengers; and on the reason for the avoidable disaster.

I owe it to the 1522 passengers, and crew, who died, as well as the 705 who survived, to offer an alternative to the official version, which makes no allowance for greed, connivance, disloyalty or treachery; offering only heroism and typical British, and American, true-grit as a basis for its morale. I would like to stress this is a work of fiction, which highlights the questions raised, and is not intended to offer the final solution to what occurred. That I have taken some liberties with history, and the facts, I have no doubt, but the narrative is concerned with people rather than explicit detail or logistics.

The real truth will never be learned until the *Titanic* is raised - which is not likely - but my version seems, to me at least, as probable as the official one.

Paul Brooke
Lancing, Sussex.
March 1994.

THE FIRST DAY

Declan Reilly leaned on the long-handled shovel in a moment's respite from the back-breaking labour he was engaged upon. It was stiflingly hot in the Boiler-Room despite the April chill which enshrouded the ship, outside, beyond the thick, steel plates of the hull. His rugged features were stained with coal-dust, like an army of blackheads on the march, except where rivulets of sweat, leaking from underneath the unruly mop of thick, black hair, had cut channels through the grime on his face and neck. He was one of the "black gang"; a stoker; the lowest of the low aboard the pride of the White Star Line's fleet, but that fact did not bother the inherently cheerful Declan one little bit: it was not something which worried him. He did his job, took his money, and to hell with the rest of them!

The circular boiler towered above him, as tall as a two-storied house, and the hungry fire in its belly winked at him through the square hole which was its ravenous mouth. It was insatiable; demanding; a strength-sapping mistress. He could feel the blast of its heat on his face and he plucked a dirty rag from his back pocket, easing the fire-door shut with it, to save his fingers. The dampers were fully open, causing a roaring sound deep in Boiler No 5, as the blaze struggled to convert water into steam to power the gigantic, 50,000 horsepower reciprocating engine, which in due course would drive the shafts to turn the three enormous screws in the stern of the ship. None of this overawed Declan; he had seen it all before over many years of service as man and boy.

He mopped his brow with a soiled cloth, no thought of hygiene in his mind: he was dirty already, in the middle of his shift, so what harm would a little more dirt do now. Declan was twenty-eight, and had been at sea for twelve years; a lowly stoker for all of that time, with no thought of promotion: just another 'thick paddy' as far as his ship-mates were concerned.

Though affable enough, he was a man of quiet intelligence, not given to sharing any part of himself with other men. Let them think what they liked about him: he cared not for their approbation. He did his job for a purpose, banked his wages, and minded his own business. Pretty soon now he would have sufficient capital for his dream: a small-holding on the west coast of Ireland, enough for a wife and his quota of children - if God willed it - far, far away from the trouble which was coming. He was a gentle man, a pacifist, and wanted no part of Irish Nationalism. What he wanted now was his bunk and the bottle of Bushmills he had hidden under his pillow. He wiped the back of his hand across his dry lips. Yes, that was the part of Ireland he wanted most at this moment!

Declan was by no means workshy, and knew just what liberties he could take without pushing his foreman, Leading Stoker Williams, too far. Taff Williams was a taciturn individual, a Company man not given to the sort of childish frivolity which affected his gang: the horse play and banter which kept them fresh in a mindless, unrewarding job. Declan knew, from his wealth of experience, the exact moment his charge would need feeding again; like an anxious mother with a newborn infant needing constant sustenance. He stood up off the shovel and opened the fire-door to check. A blast of heat caught him on the face: the fire was glowing white-hot: it was time for a feed. He banged the door shut and moved to the forward coal bunker. He knew his job without Williams having to remind him constantly, like the Leading Hand had to do with most of the other stokers - Taff was a stickler for having things done right - and the value of balancing his supply of coal, some from this bin and some from that, so it was consumed at an even rate. A little thought now, at the beginning of the voyage, could save a deal of hard work later on. Declan opened the door to the bunker and recoiled from a rush of acrid fumes which assaulted his senses: making him cough and splutter, and causing his tear-ducts to run. He slammed the door shut and secured it with the hinged locking-bars which made it watertight.

The Irishman was not one to panic: he had seen the like before. Some little spark from the boiler's inferno, or a welder's torch, had found its way amongst the coal. The boilers had been fired up, and modifications, and the easing of stiff, new fittings, had been going on for several days: ever since the ship left Southampton on her maiden voyage, and before. The tiny gleam of fire had done its work on the tinder-dry fuel, feeding off the oxygen provided by the constantly opening portal. Now a section of the garnered coal was alight and smouldering in the dark recesses of the bunker. No obvious flame or glow showed in the murky interior. Declan permitted himself a few moments to recover before setting off in search of the Leading Stoker. He found Williams in No 3 Boiler-Room, berating an idler.

"The ship's supposed to get across the Atlantic, boyo," the Welshman was saying. "At the rate you're going, we won't get steam up in this boiler until we reach New York!" The stoker, under the lash of William's tongue, made a gorgon face at the Leading Hand's back as he turned away to face the distraction. Williams was a big man, of about forty years, from the Rhondda Valley. He had spent half his working life mining coal, until he broke away from the sullied cwm with its interminable slag-heaps and depressive flavour, and the other half dealing with its consumption: always in the bowels of the earth, or a ship, away from the light. He was pasty-faced and asthmatic as a result of a lifetime spent breathing canned air, or displayed the beginnings of silicosis from the continual coal dust in the air.

"Taff, yer better cum an' take a look," Declan suggested unobtrusively, never one to shout his mouth off unless he was in drink.

"What's up?" inquired Williams.

"Yer best cum," insisted Declan and said no more. Although he had not served with the Irishman long, Williams already knew he was not a chancer, like most of the men on the shift, and had awarded him some grudging respect: Reilly was not likely to make a fuss over nothing.

"Get your finger out," Williams snapped at the errant stoker. "We sail in a couple of hours: get that boiler up to pressure," and then followed in the wake of the retreating Irishman.

"I can't see anything," complained Williams, peering into the gloom of the bunker, from am awkward, bending stance. This was not doing his back any good.

"Oi till yer, oi saw a poof o' smoke an' caught a whiff o' gas: yer wouldn't be makin' oop a ting loike dat, now would yers? Dere's a foire in dere, oi'm tilling yer," protested Declan. Williams straightened up, rubbing the arch of his back with a spare hand.

"No, Dec, I don't think you made it up." He slammed the door shut. "We'll give it a few minutes to cook up again."

They chatted, while they waited, about the sumptuousness of the ship they were on; about the likelihood of its reported invincibility; about the effect it would have on the world when it had proved its worth. One thing they agreed upon: all this would avail them nothing apart from a pittance of a wage and a steady job.

"Well, let's take another look, boyo," suggested Williams when he judged the time was right; opening the steel door cautiously, as if he expected a rush of flame or worse. When nothing came forth, he stepped into the opening and sniffed, like a tracker dog testing the air, and then he coughed uncertainly, affectedly.

"I think you're right, Dec," he admitted. "I caught a definite whiff of something there." Williams shut the door hurriedly and put the locking-bars back in place. "Look you, I'm gowin' to find the Second Engineer, see. You stay yere an' don't let anyone open this door until I get back... oh... and mind you don't go tellin' anybody 'bout it neither, see. It could be awkward: veeery awkward, boyo," he maintained.

"Sure, but yer should know me by now, Taff," admonished Declan. The Leading Stoker grinned at him uncharacteristically.

"I'm sure I dooo," he agreed, and went off in the general direction of the Engine-Room. Both men understood the seriousness of the problem.

The Royal Mail Ship *Titanic* lay off Queenstown, near Belfast, close to where she was born in the shipyard of Harland and Wolff, with her sister-ship *Olympic*; returning like a fully fledged young, steel monolith, to visit the parents who spawned her. The tenders which serviced her, supplying last minute provisions, ferrying out passengers and visitors, were dwarfed by her sheer hulk as they came alongside her entry port to offer up their cargoes. A marvel of engineering and construction techniques, she was the largest man-made object in the world at the time - 882ft long, 92ft across the beam, 97ft in depth and weighing 45,000 tons - along with the *Olympic*, and her baby sister *Britannia,* already under fabrication at Harland and Wolff. They were the first of the super-ships which would come, one day, to rule the oceans of the world - Isambard Kingdom Brunel's principles finally proved - palaces lavishly decorated and equipped, to give their clients the regal feeling which dominates the minds of the rich and famous as they venture abroad: the experience alone creating some sort of special status in the eyes of the not so fortunate. So vast were they on their proportions, these ships, no one really expected these monstrosities, made of heavy steel plate, to even float, but when they did, took on the mantle of invincibility, championed by the owners and media alike - it was a good story; it sold both berths and newspapers! Their futuristic design fuelled the stories. The *Titanic was* divided into watertight compartments which could be shut off from one another, to keep them dry: like the segments of a tangerine, part of the whole but separate entities, protected by the rind; each a little world of its own. The configuration allowed four, maybe five, of these divisions to be flooded, but no more, before the ship was in danger of sinking. No circumstances had been imagined where this would be the case. From this misinformation, the myth of the *Titanic's* invulnerability came: the notion that man had, at last, conquered the elements in which he lived with his ingenuity: that nothing could hurt or threaten her. It was good for business, and for the White Star Line, and International Mercantile Marine which owned the Company.

The Chairman of the White Star Line was on board. He was making the voyage for two reasons: to show confidence in the vessel for which he was responsible and to have a well earned rest, a reward for the traumas he had recently experienced. He was just fifty years of age; a high-flyer who had come a long way in his short life; admitted to partnership, in the Line, in 1891, and elected Chairman twelve years later on the death of his father. The super-liners, the Olympic Class, had been his brain-child, and he had seen them through from inception to fruition. The object of the exercise was to steal the Atlantic luxury passenger trade from the Cunard Line, and then who knows what? The sky was the limit if they were a success; the Indian and Pacific Ocean trade from the Union Castle Line; the Ellerman and Bucknell Line, perhaps? The White Star Line would be the only way to travel for the discerning voyager. The aircraft was seen as a laughable toy for rich men, at the time; its potential, or threat, not yet foreseen.

The *Olympic* had made her maiden voyage in June 1911. It was a triumph! Now it was the *Titanic's* turn, and the hype had begun all over again. The maiden voyage had originally been set for 20th March, of this year, but disaster struck: the *Olympic* was badly damaged in a collision with the Royal Navy Cruiser *Hawke*, her hull stove in. The *Titanic's* voyage was delayed due to the necessity of diverting services and materials to repair her sister-ship. The dent to the White Star Line's reputation was far worse than a few broken sheets of steel plate aboard the *Olympic* - their competitors capitalised on it - and all of the Chairman's resourcefulness was needed for this repair job. He had enlisted the help of all his friends in Fleet Street, and called in some favours owed, to bolster up the myth. He had the revised sailing time announced in "The Times", 10th April 1912. This time nothing must be allowed to go wrong: his presence on board was to ensure it: it needed a hands-on approach. Even so, the response for berths was not as good as it should have been; and to make things look right, several of the other White Star Line's sailings were cancelled, the passengers being transferred to the *Titanic*.

At the cocktail party in his luxury stateroom, taking place while the ship prepared for sea, the Chairman's fears were only just beginning to be assuaged as he calculated the quality of his guests, passengers all. Once the vessel reached New York, the rapidly tarnishing reputation of the Line would be ready for polishing up again. The American Financier who owned the Company should be well pleased! Most of the talk, at the party, was about the ship: several of the party-goers were the Chairman's friends, all anxious to give him their support.

"Well, I think she's a topping ship," complimented an English Lord, here by personal invitation of the Chairman: an image-booster. "Damn fine, don't you agree, m'dear?" His wife, a successful couturier, did agree but she was busy talking business to Ida Straus, the wife of Isador, the owner of Macy's in New York, the largest department store in the world.

"It should be," broadcast the Chairman, for all the guests to hear, "it cost us a small fortune to bring it to the splendour you see before you." Colonel John Jacob Astor was present in the close knot around the Chairman, with his young wife, Madeline, and Benjamin Guggenheim, the ageing playboy son of the mining and smelting family, who was always in thick of things at parties. Isador Straus was obsessed with the cost of the fittings and the equipment.

"Perhaps you should have come to see me," he confided to the Chairman, "I would have made you a better price." He guffawed at his own little joke, and his wife glared at him, disapprovingly, lovingly.

"I hear the Vanderbilts are not coming," Ida remarked to the English Lady, trying to cover up what she saw as her husband's gaff in this company - not that it appeared to worry Isador unduly.

"No, I understand they cancelled at the last minute, though apparently, their luggage is still aboard."

"They should worry about their luggage," offered Isador, not content to be suppressed, "they can afford to have luggage all around the world."

"Ah well, she doesn't care for us, anyhow," commented the plump Ida wistfully. "I'm sure the voyage will be very pleasant without them." The Countess of Rothes joined in the conversation. They were a privileged lot, and the Chairman was pleased to have them aboard. Their recommendation, of the *Titanic*, would speak volumes: much, much more than hackneyed advertising.

"I suppose you will be taking a shot at the Blue Riband?" inquired the Lord.

"Sadly, not on this trip. We must nurture the engines; see what they are capable of before we make the attempt. However, in the future, it would be satisfying to wear the Riband on our Company pennant," explained the Chairman.

He tugged at his moustache and then twirled one of the waxed ends with his fingers, a nervous habit he did not like, and stopped himself from doing it before anyone noticed. He glanced around to see if anybody had seen him, and his eyes fell on the Second Officer, who had entered the suite. The officer approached him nervously, obviously out of place amid this gathering, full of affluent people with elegant clothes.

"Excuse me, sir," he began quietly, conspiratorially.

"Yes, yes, what is it?" demanded the Chairman, annoyed at the intrusion.

"The Captain's compliments, sir. He wonders if you could spare him a few moments of your time."

"Where is he?"

"On the bridge, sir." The Chairman sighed. He had not expected to be at the Captain's beck and call.

"What is the pro..." he began, and then noticed the officer was shaking his head, and thought better of finishing the question. He looked at the young officer long and hard: the man stared back impassively, inscrutability.

"I understand it is important, sir... or he would not be bothering you a time like this," encouraged the Second Officer diplomatically.

"Yes, of course," acknowledged the Chairman. "I will come at once. Wait there; I will be with you in a moment." The Chairman looked for an excuse to cover his absence from his own party; not the done thing in this sort of company.

The Captain paced up and down on the bridge, ignoring the Chief Engineer who waited nearby. He was getting too old to face these sort of problems any more. There had been a time when he had relished them but not any longer: he was sick of the sea: these newfangled ships were becoming too complicated, and ungainly, for a man who had started his sea-time in the glorious age of sail. All he wanted out of life now was to get this deadweight to New York, then he could retire and enjoy his grandchildren. He was a short, stocky man, aged in the service of the Company, with a trim, snowy, naval beard, and the deep lines of long experience etched into his weather-beaten face. His intelligent features radiated quiet authority; backed up by the four, broad gold rings on each sleeve of his uniform coat; and the respect he had earned during his time at sea went before him wherever he travelled. The clear, blue eyes missed nothing. He did not like this command. He had been in control of the *Olympic* at the time of the collision, but it was not really his fault. These ships went so fast and took so long to stop, they could be almost unmanageable at times: they were so heavy and ponderous in their handling, no Master could expect to be adept in such a short space of time. He had narrowly avoided another disaster at Southampton, when the stern of the *New York* had come within four feet of the *Titanic,* as she passed at the outset of her passage to America, by way of Cherbourg and Belfast, and he realised then he wanted out of this awesome responsibility as soon as possible. However, with this voyage over, it would be someone else's problem: he would be ensconced in his retirement. He had conducted handling exercises between leaving Cherbourg and arriving here, in the Irish Sea, and knew a little more about the *Titanic's* behaviour than he knew before, but he would never learn it all in the time he had left; only the few, short days until New York was reached. His successor would have to learn his own lessons!

The latest news had not been very welcome. The accident in the *Olympic*, while under his command, had not been the diadem to crown the long, distinguished career of the White Star Line's senior captain, and here was another incident to frustrate him, under the nose of the Chairman, and the ship's replacement designer; as if the Gods of the Sea were thumbing their noses at him in the dying moments of an illustrious passage through life, and because he had survived everything they had thrown at him. Whatever was wrong, it would be his fault: the buck always stopped with the captain, and he was not used to having the supreme authority, of the Company which employed him, overlooking his shoulder. For far too long he had been God when he stood on the bridge of his ship. Perhaps he could get out of this awful responsibility for once: if delay was inevitable, let it be at the Chairman's behest: the Captain was too wearied by life to want the worry any longer.

The Chairman appeared on the bridge, closely followed by the Second Officer. He looked somewhat irate, and was blowing hard from a stiff climb up the companionway. The Captain stopped in mid-stride and hurried over, anxious to forestall any outburst in front of the officers and crew present: the Chairman was a person of uncertain temper.

"'I have a function in progress," he complained as he confronted the Captain. "What the devil is going on?" The Captain looked him straight in the eye, without any hint of conciliation.

"Good of you to come, sir. I won't keep you for more than a few minutes."

"It is a trifle inconvenient," the Chairman continued to bemoan, "I have some eminent people waiting on me." The Captain looked around him ambivalently.

"Shall we go outside?" he suggested, indicating the winged-bridge, overlooking the Irish mainland, which failed to impress the Chairman.

"If you have anything to say, for God's sake! Get on with it! I must get back to my guests." The Captain shrugged: he had tried his best to keep this quiet. Even so, he moved to position himself between the rest of the company and the Chairman, as if hoping to absorb the sound of their voices and prevent anything palpable from reaching the eager ears of his juniors.

"There is a fire on board in the forrard coal bunker of No 5 Boiler-Room," he declared. The Chairman looked at him askance.

"You don't need my help to put it out, do you? Deal with it, man!" The Captain sighed: this was not a helpful attitude.

"I'm afraid it's not as simple as that. It will take time," he informed the Chairman circumspectly.

"What do you mean... 'time'?"

"Twenty-fours hours or so: maybe longer. It all depends how bad things are down there."

"Twenty-fours hours to put out a fire!" The Chairman was incredulous.

"There are hundreds of tons of coal in that bunker," explained the Captain patiently. "It will have to be cleared out, the fire dealt with, and then refilled: twenty-four hours at least, depending on how hard I can get the black-gang to work. It need not delay us more than two days." The Captain had erred on the conservative side: he was not in the business of making imprudent promises.

"Delay the voyage! Are you mad? There will be no delay!" insisted the Chairman.

"We cannot go to sea with a fire in our belly!" contested the Captain. The two men glared at each other, horns locked, like immovable rams squaring up in an argument over territory.

"After the *Olympic's* collision, the Company's reputation is already at rock bottom: we are a laughing stock in the shipping world. I do recall you had something to do with that, Captain! It has been a hard enough job to fill the ship's berths as it is, and we are still short of passengers. Another delay... any delay... will make us look downright incompetent. We must sail on time, as advertised... without fail." The Chairman was adamant: the Captain was equally unyielding.

"I am responsible for the safety of this ship: we cannot sail with a fire on board: it is potentially dangerous. I would also suggest we clear the ship while the necessary work is carried out."

"Now I am sure you are going mad!" stormed the Chairman. "Clear the ship indeed! His voice carried to the officers, on the bridge, who looked away in embarrassment, pretending not to hear. "And what do you think that will do for our prestige?... This fire is raging below, is it?"

"No, but it is smouldering," the Captain had to admit. The Chairman clutched at the slender straw.

"Ah... smouldering is it now? Not a real fire at all."

"It could burst into flame at any moment, and with the amount of coal involved, it could be extremely hazardous." The Captain did not care to be ridiculed in front of his crew; his lofty station belittled. "It must be put out now, whatever the delay; and whatever the damage to your public image." The Chairman looked around for an ally, and spotted the Chief Engineer, waiting on the sidelines.

"And what do you say, Chief: can this... fire... be contained?" The Chief Engineer had his own career to consider: he was much younger than the Master of the *Titanic*. To have achieved his present position, he must be regarded as at the top of the marine-engineering tree: a commission he did not wish to jeopardise.

"If we sprayed the coal with water and then battened down the bulkhead door, to starve the fire of oxygen, I think we might well reach New York safely, and discharge our passengers without serious consequence." He voiced his considered verdict and then flashed a tentative glance, full of contrite apology, at his Captain: he would never know just how relieved the Master was to have this responsibility taken away from him.

The Chairman turned on the Captain.

"What do you think?" he asked.

"You already know what I think, sir. We should evacuate the ship and put out the fire. However, if we do as the Chief suggests, it is true, we might make our destination without serious occurrence. I am only an employee, after all, so I shall leave the final decision to you. I shall do as I am instructed... as I have always done." The Captain turned away and took a sudden, special interest in the binnacle.

The Chairman examined the faces around him, the Second Officer, the Chief Engineer, seeking inspiration. What should he do for the best?

"What is the fuel situation? Can we reach New York without using this coal bunker?" he inquired.

"Certainly," agreed the Chief Engineer. "We have more than enough coal. It is just a matter of logistics, really, moving coal about to suit ourselves, balancing up the rest of our supply... we can't have one boiler running out of fuel while the rest have plenty, can... "

"Quite." The Chairman considered the position for a few moments longer. "Well that settles it, then," he announced, looking to attract the Captain's attention; attempting to justify himself. "I am sorry, but too much time and effort, and money of course, has been spent on this endeavour: there can be no further delay." He turned back to the Chief Engineer. "You will do as you said: douse down that coal and batten down that bunker."

"Aye, aye, sir."

"Good, good! Of course, it goes without saying, I don't want any word of this to leak out." The two officers nodded gravely. When he realised the Captain's back was still turned, the Chairman made the point of including him in the dialogue. "Captain, who else knows about this?" The Master turned back to face the gathering; he looked worried.

"Well, Mister?" he demanded of the Chief Engineer.

"Us four, sir; my number two; Leading Stoker Williams; and the stoker who found the fire."

"Keep it that way, will you," chipped in the Chairman, "even if you have to grease a few palms. This sort of thing is likely to cause panic if it gets out, and I am not having that sort of thing on this voyage. Gentleman, the *Titanic* will arrive, on time, off the Statue of Liberty, in under six days, as publicised. We shall proceed with all speed on this passage, as a test run: I want the Blue Riband hanging from the Company Pennant before the end of the year."

"Yes, sir," chorused the two officers. The Captain was not so enthusiastic, or forthcoming, but then it was no longer his responsibility.

Three families joined the *Titanic,* off Queenstown, on that fateful day; all transferred from other sailings, and all very different. Two were quite happy with the change but one was not.

David Peacock and his wife, Molly, were well pleased with their First Class stateroom. They were used to opulence, and grandeur, having travelled to various parts of the world by ship. David was a Director of the de Vere Wool Company, of the City of London, in charge of new markets, and was on his way to investigate the New World as a possible source of fresh business for his traditional firm. He came from the suburbs of London, the rich end of Forest Hill where the community was advantaged, and was used to the good things in life. The wool trade was booming, especially in Germany, where the Kaiser was preparing for war, and equipping his troops in new uniforms made of merino wool, largely imported from South Africa, which was a hard-wearing and economical material. The Peacocks had brought their children with them on this trip, a boy and a girl, but they would not be encumbered with them on the voyage, which they regarded as a second honeymoon. The children were lodged with their nanny, in a cabin in the Second Class portion of the ship: out of sight and out of mind until they were wanted. They were combining business with pleasure; taking a holiday when work was completed, and the children would be kept in their place, and under strict control, for the duration of their stay. For the time being, they were quite prepared to be fêted, and indulged, at the firm's expense before they had to bear the cost of their vacation, which they could well afford.

Thomas Pirbright had staked everything he had on a gamble. He was going to America to join his brother. Tom was a journeyman carpenter but his brother, Albert, was a very clever fellow, well versed in the installation of electricity, the new marvel of the age. The two brothers had decided, some time before when their parents died, that the New World was the Land of Golden Opportunity, where England lacked the urgency which would bring them a fortune. Millions of homes in the States invited conversion to the innovative, invisible power which was ready to spread its tentacles across the globe; while the staid English still regarded it with suspicion and distrust. A fortune was waiting to be made, or so Bert believed, and he had sold up his dead parents' home, and his own, to take the plunge; to scout the lie of the land; to set up a business in a healthier pecuniary climate; to take maximum advantage of a beckoning opportunity. Now it had all been achieved. They were set fair to clean up, and it was time for Tom to join his brother who was armed with contracts. A great number of the properties were constructed of clapboard, so Tom would supervise the preparation of the woodwork and leave Bert to sweep in, and out, with a minimum of delay, to install the wiring and fittings. They had several years' worth of guaranteed work and Bert bad already recruited a local workforce to help them. Tom had sold up his own home, and effects, and was on his way to New York, to be reunited with Bert, bringing with him Amy, his wife, and their three children, and his sister-in-law, Clara, Bert's wife, and her two sons. They were travelling steerage, or Third Class, to conserve their resources, and were almost overwhelmed to cruise in this great ship, and if not in luxury, at least in good company.

Only Jonathan Wainwright was not a happy man at the sudden change of his arrangements, if not for his own sake, but for the sake of his wife, Lorna. She was not pleased at having been transferred to the *Titanic,* with her husband and children, for she had a presentiment of doom about the voyage, which had assailed her as soon as she set foot on the deck. She would not have sailed if she had any choice in the matter but there was no other way to keep to her husband's strict timetable, which allowed no variance. Jonathan was a Professor of Science and was on his way to take up a Chair in an American University, for which he was already late, and would brook no further delay in case it damaged his future prospects. He was a very practical man, and a firm disbeliever in such things as portents but was stuck with his wife's auguries of disaster and destruction, nonetheless, in which she was more than vocal. Even the sumptuousness of the Second Class cabin had not assuaged her fears, just as the solidity of the huge hull seemed to compound them.

"I really do not feel safe," Lorna complained, as the Wainwrights unpacked their cases, and Jonathan was exasperated.

"I cannot see why, dear. This ship is reputed to be the safest vessel afloat. It was designed by the greatest of talents, constructed by the finest of builders from the best available materials, to the highest specification and safety standards, and crewed by the most experienced of sailors. I cannot, for the life of me, see what you need to fear: the White Star Line has a marvellous reputation and a wonderful safety record or I would not have booked with them in the first place." Lorna was well used to her husband's logical approach to life, but her strange feelings would not go away. The ship, despite its gilded fittings and rare grandeur, was a dark, forbidding monstrosity in the recesses of her mind. The hairs on the nape of her neck were in a constant condition of movement, and her nerves had tingled in morbid anticipation of some terrible happenstance, at every moment since she first set foot on the solid deck. She gathered her young daughters in her arms, attempting to garner some comfort from them.

"I don't care what you say, John," she demurred, "I cannot help my feelings. Something terrible is going to happen to this ship; I can sense it in my bones. Can we, please, wait for another ship?"

"Don't be ridiculous!" snapped the irate Jonathan, "you will frighten the children". Then his tone changed abruptly, and he became consolatory. "Look old girl, you know I must take up my appointment in a week and that it has already been put back once. If we wait for another ship, the University will probably cable me to say "Don't bother to come at all". You know how long I've waited for this chance. America is the crucible of modern science, full of inventiveness, innovation and with the capital to exploit new discoveries. I want to be... eh... we agreed I should be part of such a process, did we not? You'll see, when we arrive in New York, safe and sound, you will laugh about all this. You are being silly, really, my love."

"Have you considered that if you do not wait for another ship, you might never arrive at the University at all, let alone be part of this modern revolution you are always talking about?" persisted the unhappy wife.

"For God's sake! Lorna! What can I say to convince you nothing is going to happen to this damn ship?" roared Jonathan. "It is a floating castle, an ocean fortress which nothing can touch. Don't you understand, the ship contains watertight compartments: it is unsinkable; invincible? Don't you think I should know? God himself would be hard put to deal it a mortal blow!" Jonathan was an atheist: he dealt in facts not fanciful ideas.

"Don't you think that might be pushing God a little too far?" snapped Lorna. Her husband snorted in reply.

Taff Williams came back into the boiler-room with a supercilious grin on his face. He felt important, proud to be part of a loyal conspiracy to avert a "storm in a teacup", as the situation had been described by the Second Engineer. Declan Reilly was going about his business unconcerned, stoking the hungry boiler.

"Dec, leave that," ordered Williams. "Fix up a hose to the hydrant. We are going to douse the fire in the bunker."

"A fat lot 'o good that'll do," advised Declan. "We don't know fir sure how bad de foire has taken hould. Twould be batter to clear... "

"Orders is orders, boyo," disputed Williams. "We are to douse the coal and then batten down the bunker. Look you, if we doo as we are told, without argument, see, there will be a few quid in it for us: a loooverly bonus like, eh." The Irishman shrugged.

"It's a f-hookin' risk ye're takin', Taff! Annie-ting kin happen if you's don't put de foire out," admonished Declan.

"Nothing is gowin' to happen, see, boy. The Chief says the bunker is airtight, and if we batten it down, we will starve the fire of oxygen, and it will go out." Declan looked confused: he did not know about such things: a fire was a fire, to him, and should be put out properly.

"Oi don't loike de sounda dat," he complained.

"Well, you'll just have to trust me, see... me and the Chief Engineer," Williams pronounced pompously. "It's alright, Dec, you don't have to worry: the Chief knows what he's dooin'. Yoo just have to keep quiet 'bout this, see; doo what you're told and yoo'll get your bonus. Do yoo understand?" Declan nodded his head. "Good boy," lauded Williams. "You're in for a bit of overtime tooo. This Boiler-Room is out of bounds for the duration of the voyage; to any of the crew, apart from the officers. They be wanting yoo too doo a twelve hour shift, each day, till we reach New York. Yoo can manage that, can't yoo?"

"'It's a wunder dey don't wants to make it twenty-fours hours a f-hooking day," submitted Declan sarcastically.

"Don't fret yourself, boyo: I'll be dooin' the other twelve hours; just you and me, see, 'til we make port. Just think of the money, Dec, and hold your tongue. It'll make it easier for all of us." Declan Reilly hawked and spat on the deck: he was not impressed!

The *Titanic* sailed from Belfast exactly on time, according to schedule, being accorded the adulation reserved for any great ship on her maiden voyage. The ship's orchestra played lively tunes of the day, from a prominent position on the Boat Deck, and the excited passengers crowded the rails to experience the tremendous send off. Ships anchored in the Roads, and the *Titanic's* attendants and handmaidens, blew long blasts on their sirens and foghorns as the megalith gathered way. Streamers trailed from the Promenade Deck, down the sheer sides of the ship; bedecked as she already was with fluttering, windswept bunting and a profusion of flags. She was a grand sight to the crowd of onlookers lining the shore for a sight of the liner in motion; the curious, the enthusiasts, and many of the workers who built her, had come to see the culmination of their handiwork in glorious mobility.

The *Titanic* turned northwest into the North Channel, after clearing Whitehead, and came up to half-ahead as she cruised past the Mull of

Kintyre, and on towards Islay and the open sea. Many of the passengers stayed on deck, as it was a clear day, and the wonderful sights of the Scottish Isles were plainly visible; the lush, variegated foliage of the evergreen trees, tan, emerald, olive and sage; the grassy valleys and bare rocks; and the snow-clad peaks of the Paps of Jura rose up out of the land like the stunning adornments of a well endowed woman. Clear of the land, the ship turned southwest and set a course for Cape Race, in Newfoundland, leaving the Scottish Mainland, the Western Isles, the Orkneys and Shetlands, and Muckle Flugga, the most northern of the British Isles, directly in her wake. She came up to full-ahead and set off across the Atlantic Ocean at a good speed.

With nothing to look at, except the receding land, which became more and more indistinct as the liner sailed on, the passengers began to drift away from the rails; back to their cabins to complete unpacking; or to go in search of further distractions, and delights, which had not yet been discovered. Far below in the depths of the ship, the crew began, what would be to them, several days of hard graft in order to keep the voyagers happy, in varying degrees, according to how much they had paid, and what status they held in the class-ridden, pretentious society that made up the *Titanic's* current population.

In the depths of No 5 forward coal bunker, the obstinate fire refused to succumb to the deluge of water, which had pervaded it, or the starvation of air it had suffered. Under tons of coal, it clung to life, inhibited by the dampness all around, but nourished by little pockets of oxygen trapped in the nooks and crannies of the piled up fuel. It could not burst into flame, so was it constrained, but it glowed dimly in the complete, jet darkness; fastening hold of any chance it could take to extend. As it smouldered, it dried out the coal alongside and moved on, infecting the unburned fuel with its purpose; to escape from the submerged dungeon which tried to hold it dormant. Gradually it spread its tentacles outwards and upwards seeking its final destiny.

Possibly only one family was not involved, in some way, with the *Titanic's* leaving of her home port - although she was registered in Liverpool, and carried that name high on her stern. Lorna

Wainwright could not raise any enthusiasm for the pomp and ceremony which accompanied the event, and stayed in her cabin with the children. Her only interest, like that of the Captain, was to get to New York as soon as possible and be done with the strange feelings which plagued her. Jonathan was pleased that they were at last under way, and was naturally interested in the machinations of the vessel because of his calling, but his elation was overshadowed by his wife's depressive mood and he stayed in the cabin with her, missing all the fun. He had several papers to peruse, before he took up his new post, and he had brought any number of scientific journals to read on the voyage. He would keep himself occupied with them.

He would have much preferred a wife who would have joined in the spirit of things - her attitudes frustrated him at times - but he loved her dearly: she was the mother of his darling daughters and she was the right type of women for a man, of his ilk, to have at his side. She was a perfect hostess, and domestic manager, with a temperament well suited to his type of life: she could hold her own in sensible, and serious, conversation with any of his colleagues or peers. She was an English rose, peachy cheeked and delicately featured, with long brown hair which was always neatly groomed. She was the sort of woman you could take anywhere and she would fit in, look at home and act accordingly without ever being an embarrassment. She could cope with any situation calmly, however fraught, and was a definite asset. However, all types of perfection have their blemishes, and she was no exception. When she got a bee in her bonnet, as she had now, it was unshakeable, no matter what was said to her and how hard anyone tried to assuage her fears. It was not that she was inclined to show anyone up - she kept her qualms within her own family circle - but Jonathan was an intolerant man, and could not see how anyone, let alone his rational wife, could hold such pedantic views when the weight of evidence was diametrically opposed to their point of view.

For the time being, he would humour her, accepting she was naturally frightened by the sheer size of the ship, and its ungainly movement, but when they arrived in New York, he intended to remind her frequently of how silly her fears had been and how she had ruined the exciting voyage for him, in the hope it might prevent any future manifestation of her misgivings, and leave him to enjoy a peaceful life. In deference to her feelings, he would stay with her while she was awake, leaving the cabin only to take meals in the Dining-Room, and reserve his expeditions of exploration on the ship for a time when she slept, if only fitfully. He would come to wander the decks at night, examining this and that - any of the ship's functions, or apparatus, that took his interest - to salve his disappointed life-force that was naturally curious about anything out of the ordinary, or futuristic. In this way he hoped to keep the peace with Lorna - she was demanding of his company in her current state of mind; seeming to garner strength from him to face her imagined ordeal - and salvage what he could from what should have been a mind-boggling experience for him.

The Marconi-Room was already becoming busy. There was a flurry of cablegrams to be sent, to all parts of the globe, by the rich who liked to play with the new found convenience of wireless telegraphy. Most of the cables were meaningless expressions of joy, at being encased in the sumptuousness of the *Titanic,* sent to impress less fortunate friends and relatives, but there were some business communications from passengers who could run their empires from abroad.

The Radio Operators, Harold Bride and Jack Phillips, were not members of the crew, and did not come into the ship's chain of command. They were employees of the Marconi Company and were required to operate a commercial venture which would prove the reliability of wireless telegraphy to the influential passengers aboard, as well as earn good money for the firm. Any messages sent to the ship, for the attention of the Captain and his Officers, must wait their turn to be delivered, depending on how busy the operators were, as the liner was considered to be well capable of voyaging without the aid of newfangled inventions, as most ships had up to this point in time. The radio was a desirable luxury, not an essential one.

However, wireless communication was in its infancy and, despite its serious, practical side, was still an enthusiast's plaything to be experimented on to find the true bounds of its ultimate application. Radio's impact on the age was not underestimated by its champions, but a more sceptical business world, and the general public, had yet to be fully convinced. This was also part of the Radio Operators' brief; to show this type of communication was invaluable to all. Harold Bride and Jack Phillips, therefore, would experiment as much as possible during the voyage. While they were still in range of the

British Isles, they would continue to send messages to the stations on the mainland, to be transmitted from post to post until they arrived at their varied destinations. Once out of range, the message-sending would almost cease; only missives of real importance being transmitted. This would involve a great deal of sifting and selection, weeding-out and commercial favouritism, to separate the vital from the detritus: Ida Strauss's trivial communiqué to a relative would be considered much more worthwhile than Jonathan Wainwright's message of reassurance to his new employers! These consequential messages would be transmitted to other ships, in range, who carried a radio, to be passed on from ship to ship across the Atlantic, while the operators were well prepared to offer the same service from the *Titanic*. It was a time of innovation and inventiveness for them, and the process would occupy a great deal of time, and provide excitement and satisfaction.

Messages would continue to pile up in the Marconi Room, awaiting the time when the Radio Station at Cape Race was in range, and inevitably, because of the situation, efficiency would go by the board. Bride and Phillips would act in the interests of their employers pre-eminently, which would not always be in the best interests of the ship.

To the Peacocks, the liner was a labyrinth of delights. After checking the children were comfortable in the care of their nanny, they set forth to explore the ship. The *Titanic* had sailed at 1.30 pm, so there was a whole afternoon of discoveries to come before formal dinner was served. Everywhere they ventured was pristine, unspoiled by use: the heady tang of varnish and fresh paint lingered in the enclosed corridors of the lower decks of the ship. They knew there was a gymnasium, a swimming-bath and a squash racquet court but they had to be identified for future utilisation. David was ecstatic. He was a sportsman of sorts - he had played Rugby for his Public School - and liked to keep in shape to offset the extravagances of his privileged household. While Molly would not join in - raising a sweat was not her idea of a woman's role in life - she would go where she could to encourage, admire and support her husband, as that was the function she perceived for herself. David was a handsome man and her continual interest in his activities, and him, precluded any chance of his casting his eyes over other pastures. He already stood out in any crowd, with his bright, red hair flaming like a beacon to draw the gaze, so Molly felt riding herd was a sensible course to take when they ventured abroad. At home, where their life was pretty mundane, such care was not necessary. It was not that she was possessive, or had any reason to fear his continence; it was prudent to be mindful of her future security in a rapidly changing world emerging from the repression of the Victorian Era.

David and Molly could go anywhere on the ship - it was the Second and Third Class passengers whose movements were restricted - and took full advantage of their mobility, although there were certain places it would not do to be seen, such as the steerage areas. They found a Turkish Bath not noticed in the *Titanic's* brochure and moved on to the privileged precincts. They traipsed through the Writing-Room, the Lounge, the Reception-Room and the Smoking-Room, and up and down the Grand Staircase - its opulence making it the most lavish afloat. They examined the Library, the à la carte Restaurant, although the luxuriant Dining-Room would have been more than adequate for normal mortals - the Palm Court and the Veranda Café, looking for their particular niche. The Café Parisien, a reproduction of a sidewalk café where the younger set was beginning to gather, seemed to fit the bill. It offered just the sort of atmosphere the Peacocks were looking for, and were used to, and already brief acquaintances, only passed once or twice before, were on nodding terms.

Yes, decided David, these were going to be an excellent few days, with plenty of chances for immoderation, and the means to trim any inches the excesses might add to his figure! With the children out of the way, in the care of Nanny, he would have Molly entirely to himself, without the inconvenience of her usual domestic preoccupations, and he intended to use the time to revitalise his libido, which had suffered at the hands of commercialism and mercantile pressure. It was not before time for him to look to extend his progeny - large broods of children were the tradition in his family which had the means to support them - and Molly's soft body still attracted him immensely even after ten years of marriage - he never did seem to procure his fair share for some reason or another. In any case she blossomed when she was pregnant, her skin shone fair as her belly and breasts rounded out, even though she considered the whole process as a time of great inconvenience to her daily routine. Yes, she became the epitome of desire as she ripened, and David could not wait to experience the delicious ecstasy which would inaugurate the process. With this to look forward to, plus an abundance of food and drink, entertainment and enjoyment, and the pain of rigorous exercise as a catalyst to channel his sensations, this was going to be the best second honeymoon a man could wish for! Molly had no real need to worry about his steadfastness.

Thomas Andrews was another person who had the run of the ship, but his explorations were out of duty, not pleasure. He was the Managing Director of Harland and Wolff, as well as the chief among the ship's designers. He had come on the voyage as a representative of the builders, replacing Lord Pirrie, the Chairman of the shipyard in Belfast, who was in bad health and had perforce cancelled his pleasure trip, which had been at the behest of the Chairman of the White Star Line. Andrews was in an unenviable position. He had replaced the original designer, Alexander Carlisle, who had proved to be too rigid in his insistence at sticking with the initial design, which did not suit either companies involved in the construction and operation of the *Titanic*. Carlisle was a man of strong principle, inflexible, his views forcibly expressed. It was odds on he would be removed at some stage, when he came into conflict with his employers and their clients. None of this helped Andrews as he now considered he held the worst end of the stick. He would be held ultimately responsible for another man's blueprint, and whatever might go wrong would be laid at his door, while Carlisle still had the satisfaction of claiming the *Titanic* to be his own brainchild. Carlisle had not endeared himself to the White Star Line over his insistence there should be at least sixty lifeboats on the ship to carry away the passengers and crew in case of disaster. Despite the sense shown in this, it was an outrage to the Chairman, and his Board, who held the opposing view that a catastrophe was out of the question considering the amount of money which had been spent on bringing the Olympic Class of liners into service. They had a safety record second to none, and some of the most experienced sailors in the world were in control of the ships. Out-dated Board of Trade regulations insisted that only sixteen lifeboats were necessary on the ship of this passenger capacity, and while the Board of Directors excepted this as a standard, they provided an additional four collapsible boats, for safety's sake, which they considered to be adequate. Cost was not a consideration, but there was the cosmetic look of the vessel to consider, as well as the myth of invincibility, which would not be served by a further forty boats which would detract from the look of the super-liner and might engender the spectre of trepidation in some minds. Alexander Carlisle did not agree, and made his representations too unpleasantly for all involved to stomach happily. As a result he was removed from his position as Chief Designer.

Thomas Andrews felt he bore the responsibility to ensure the ship was in perfect order and he mooched about, getting in the crew's way, ensuring that all systems were go. He went everywhere; checking the Engine-Room; the boilers; the bilges in the double-bottom of the ship; the inspection tunnels alongside the giant shafts which turned the gargantuan screws. He examined every moving part from the winches in the bows to the housing for the steering gear in the stern, not entirely satisfied with anything he saw; suggesting little adjustments here and there. Like all highly technical men, he had an unfortunate manner, tunnel-vision and vehemence - although he had compromised his own principles to escape Carlisle's fate - and did not exactly enchant the officers and crew with whom he came into contact. He stole like a wraith through the bowels of the ship, always preoccupied, and pausing only to eat and sleep, as he attempted to vindicate the design he had inherited, and did not want to see go wrong in any department, for obvious reasons. At no time was he ever informed about the fire in the coal bunker, which smouldered on uninterrupted.

He had a daily meeting with the Chairman, and was quite frank in his assessments of the ship's condition. Everything was going superbly well, despite his fussiness, and he had no doubt the maiden voyage would be an unqualified success. The Chairman was more than pleased.

Thomas Andrews was not the only soul to haunt the artificial, twilight world of the lower decks. The steerage passengers lived a subterranean existence too, but not by choice. They were banned from the Promenade Deck, which was the domain of the First and Second Class passengers, and most of their amenities were several decks down. In truth their accommodation was possibly the best of its kind in any ship which plied the five oceans, for the time being, and until it deteriorated from constant, primitive abuse by the hoi-polloi - or so the Owners thought. However, they were a necessary evil for any liner, the bread and butter of the Atlantic trade, but must be kept well away from the more advantaged passengers who considered them to be "the great-unwashed". Their berths were split in two, some in the bows abaft the crew's quarters, and some in the stern just forward of the storerooms. The Third Class Dining-Room was in the centre of the ship, on Deck E which involved a considerable hike from both ends at meal-times. Their Smoke-Room was high up on the stern, and their recreation area, the Third Class Open Space, was sandwiched in between the mast which held the crows-nest and the start of the super-structure, in the fo'c'sle. It did not make for an easy life but then, to everyone else on board's satisfaction, they were out of the way, with their boorish habits, manners and practices, and out of mind. They were for the most part a motley collection of the disadvantaged from all corners of the British Isles; Irishmen from the Emerald Isle and Liverpool; Cornishmen from the West Country; Londoners; Yorkshiremen and Lancastrians; and the inevitable Scots who seemed intent on spreading their skills to every part of the globe. They sought the benefits of the New World for any number of reasons. Some travelled to join relatives; some to experience the American dream which the daily papers extolled at every opportunity; some because they were redundant in their trade or their trade itself had become superfluous; some because they were adventurous and breaks were no longer available at home; some who suffered from wanderlust; and some who perceived the clouds of war gathering over Europe and sought the isolationism of America to escape the coming holocaust. Whatever their types, or reasons, they allowed themselves to be packed in tightly like sardines, and endured the travails of their passage without complaint; all for the sake of a new, more rewarding lifestyle.

Tom Pirbright was of the adventurous type, staking his all on a dream although through Bert's groundwork, it had a sound basis - and he ventured where he was allowed on the ship in excursions of exploration, although, unbeknown to him, it was a pilgrimage to a lifestyle which he, some day, expected to gain by his efforts in America. The anorexically thin Clara and the plump Amy - ill-matched companions - did not accompany him on his wanderings. Amy's children were infants and needed much attention, constant nappy-changing, and in the baby's case, frequent breast-feeding. Clara, through her separation from Bert, had older boys, and stayed with her sister-in-law to help out, as she had no interest in the ship, apart from it being the means to reunite her with her husband, which was long overdue. Perhaps soon she could catch up in the childbearing stakes although her life would be much more complicated by it than Amy's, as she did not have the advantage of her own milk to offer an infant. On the whole, the two women existed together very well for females of the same family and to Tom's relief, did not bother him overmuch; leaving him free to follow his own interests.

With the aid of the much despised familiarity of the lower classes, Tom had soon made several casual acquaintances among his fellow, male passengers, and in the Third Class Smoking-Room, cloudy with the fug of cheap tobacco, soon found out all there was to know about them as there was not much else for the steerage passengers to do but talk. Here, in this company, there was no sign of pretentiousness, or airs and graces, and a spirit of camaraderie was forged at once. With no social barriers to overcome, and the prospect of a new life in the offing, spirits were high from the outset of the voyage. Tom soon found himself roped into, and engaged in a impromptu game of makeshift football in the open space at the bow, in which his fellow players were over-enthusiastic, and lethal, and the spectators volubly encouraging. It was a good start to a few, short days of relaxation before the hard work, awaiting him in the United States would begin. Tom was a very happy man.

The *Titanic* drove on into the deep water of the Atlantic. The weather was fine and clear: the sea calm. As the afternoon progressed into evening, the service crew prepared for dinner, in the three separate dining-rooms; the fare, and number of courses, varying according to how much each class had paid. However it was all good, wholesome food although the menus ranged from plain English to what the caterers considered to be culinary French. The sea was so flat, there were hardly any cases of seasickness reported to the Ship's Doctor, although some travellers will always feel at bit queasy before sea-legs are gained. On the whole, all the passengers enjoyed dinner and departed thereafter to pursue their interests for the rest of the evening. The orchestra started to play in the Palm Court and some passengers made their way there to be entertained. Bar-flies always head for the nearest bar, and did so; others played cards, bridge, whist and the more dangerous gambling games which men enjoy. The younger set headed for the Cafés where they could parade their finery and engage in good conversation. Others still preferred to retire early; it had been a long, exciting day. Those with children to care for would put their charges to bed and hope they would soon find sleep, to be left in the comparative safety of the cabins and storerooms by parents anxious to salvage what was left of the evening's entertainments. The hardy would take a turn around the deck, to walk off dinner, well wrapped up against the chill of the evening. The First and Second Class passengers dressed for dinner, if not in evening dress, at least in a decent suit or frock, whereas the steerage travellers wore what they had without shame. But then, they would not be seen beyond the barriers which blocked them off from the rest of the ship.

The *Titanic* was behaving well, running at about sixteen knots, with all components working correctly, much to Thomas Andrews, the Captain and the Chairman's satisfaction. She would make three hundred and eighty six miles in her first twenty-four hours. Tomorrow, she would be brought up to full ahead and kept there all day to test her cruising abilities with an almost full load; something she had not experienced before.

On Shelter Deck C, Lorna Wainwright had settled her girls into bed at a reasonable hour. They were aged nine and seven, Claire and Alice, and were normally sensible, although the splendour of dinner in unfamiliar circumstances had rather overawed them; the awe had turned to excitement, and the excitement to the inevitable bad temper and tears little girls displayed when tired out. It was not their fault, Lorna decided, and administered no castigation for their misconduct. It was the fault of this damned ship and its bizarre aura.

Jonathan was lying on his side of the bed when she returned, comfortable in his favourite cardigan, reading a scientific journal. He lifted his eyes from the lines of print and watched her as she prepared for bed. She looked tired and drawn, almost haggard, as if she had not relaxed for some time. She turned her back on him as she undressed, as if not wishing to excite him in any way, and slid into her cotton nightdress hurriedly, giving her hair a few peremptory strokes of the brush, before padding over to the bed and sliding beneath the crisp, starched sheets. She settled herself gratefully and sighed.

"Are you alright, old girl?" Jonathan inquired tenderly.

"As right as I'll ever be in this... ship," she returned.

"It will be okay, you'll see," Jonathan consoled her, beginning to pick up colloquialisms from the American couple who shared their dining table.

"Hmmmm... " was all Lorna said as she turned over and settled herself for sleep.

"The ship is going along quite nicely... and all the officers look quite happy when you see them about. That would hardly be the case if there was any problem, now would it?" Jonathan tried again to assuage her fears but she did not reply: nothing could do that.

She initiated a regular breathing rhythm in the hope her husband might think she had fallen asleep, but tired as she was, she did not want to lose consciousness. She was afraid of the horrid dreams, the psychic revelations, which might assail her. She had tried for most of the day, for Jonathan's sake, to forget her anxiety but it would not leave her. She knew how clever he was, and that he was probably talking sense, but the flesh-crawling sensation which plagued her would not go away. Yes, it was as he had said, everybody on board, she had come across, was in a joyous, holiday mood and she knew she would normally be infected herself. Happiness would not come to her; she felt lost and alone; a little island of depression in a sea of boisterousness. She berated herself, silently, for her hysteria but there was nothing much she could do about it.

Later, as she fought the eyelids which seemed determined to close, she felt Jonathan slide off the bed. Further sounds which came to her ears made her aware he was pulling on his shoes. She dared not turn around. It was not fair to cage him for her own inadequacies, and knew his spirit was inquisitive, and his mind needed stimulation, but nonetheless, when she heard the cabin door shut silently behind him, she began to whimper in her loneliness. Very soon her sobbing turned to floods of tears.

By contrast, on Bridge Deck B, Molly Peacock was taking a great deal of trouble with her bedtime deliberations. She had put away her jewellery carefully, in expensive, velvet-lined cases, and rather than clearing off the subtle make-up she applied to her face was refining it, to appear more exciting, and attractive, to her husband. David had gone to the Smoking-Room for a final cigar before retiring, and Molly was more than sure no woman would frequent the place at any time. She was aware of the heads he had turned tonight, in full view of the diners in the First Class Dining-Room, and at the Café Parisien later on, and felt very vulnerable at this moment for some strange reason. She was determined his full attention would be focused an her for the rest of the voyage, after this night. She dressed in a silk nightdress, pink and sheer, which clung to her luscious, unspoilt figure, and slipped into a matching peignoir.

She climbed into the comfortable bed and took some time arranging herself in its abundance, covering only her slender legs with the bedclothes. She organised the nightdress to show off her figure to its best advantage, hugging the flat belly and revealing just the right amount of cleavage to make herself look alluring. She spread out the peignoir around her, and settled back to wait.

David was not long. He let himself into the stateroom, hoping she was not asleep, and found her radiantly receptive. His normally rubescent complexion was flushed with the drink he had imbibed on this night of uncontrolled celebration; a heady combination of wine and spirits. A boyish grin spread across his face as he saw his wife laid out like a flower on the bed, the honey pot, cunningly veiled to excite great interest; he knew only too well what it implied. To encourage his own arousal - suffering in its intensity because of the amount he had drunk - he made his own disrobing, in Molly's full sight, a slow and deliberate affair. It was not the way he normally behaved, respecting her sensibilities, but then it was a replica honeymoon, and he had acted like this on the primary one, before Victorian morality had shaped his future conduct into a very different vein.

"Did you enjoy your cigar, dearest?" Molly inquired, a catch of anticipation in her voice. Ten years on from their wedding day she was still eminently engaging.

"Yes, it was most enjoyable," he confirmed as he stripped off his dinner jacket. "I found myself in the company of several distinguished, and interesting gentlemen. Their conversation was most elucidating. I am invited to a game of cards with them tomorrow, and I think it could put me in a favourable position with one or two of them. Their acquaintance could well provide some short-cuts to my endeavours in America. I hope you will not mind that I have agreed."

"Of course not, my love," Molly assured him, relieved his plans excluded the possibility of coming into contact with other women. "Our trip to America is principally a business one, is it not? Why should I mind?" David chortled uncharacteristically.

"Let us leave the business to New York, and in the meantime turn our attention to other considerations, shall we?"

"I am not sure I know what you mean," retorted Molly innocently, and David chuckled again. His intentions could not really be mistaken as he advanced on the bed stark naked, and Molly reached out with her arms fully extended to receive him.

"Gi' us a cuddle, gel," suggested Tom Pirbright, and then complained, "I'm cold." Amy had her amply-proportioned back towards him in the narrow confines of the steerage berth.

"We all know what vat means," Amy informed him languidly. She was tired after containing the children all day, and sluggish after the huge meal she had eaten earlier.

"C'mon, gel, I'm only arter a cuddle," Tom whinged.

"Yes, I know. It's what ya allus say. Don't ya never fink of anyfink else?"

"Wh... aaat, gel. Ya knows I love yer. What's wrong with vat?"

"Oh, go an ven, if vat's what you want. Just ya be careful, Tom Pirbright; we don't want to go starting a new life whiff me up the stick," Amy capitulated ungraciously.

"Don't worry about it, gel. We are goin' ta be able to afford loads of kids in America, so Bert says, ven we git orf the grand. We kin 'ave an English family an' an American one too, hey?"

"It's alright for 'im: 'e don't have to have va bleedin' fings," protested Amy, but nonetheless gave herself up to her husband's attentions, although she made herself available to him rather than encouraging him. He was a good man, was Tom, and she was always prepared to look after his comforts, despite her insincere protestations.

"How's it going, Dec?" Taff Williams inquired insensitively when he came to relieve the Irishman at eleven pm.

"Oi'm f-hooked. Dis ain't no joke, yer know," grumbled Declan. His skin was bathed in sweat; his uncomfortably damp clothes coated in grime. The bright red kerchief he wore around his neck to stop the perspiration running down his back had changed to a burnt-umber hue. He was not very happy.

"Stop moanin', Dec, it's only for a fue days, boy. Think of the money!" encouraged Taff, with the air of a man who had not yet had to climb this mountain of physical endurance. He would not be so cheerful when his own twelve-hour stint was over.

"Who taught of dis torture?" Declan wanted to know.

"The Chief said the orders came down from the Chairman, who's on board. You can't get orders from higher than that."

"It's a great pity he doesn't handle a shoovil himself. Oi could do wit' a hand," joked Declan.

"There's no chance of that, boyo: he's tooo busy drinkin' champagne an' havin' a good time to worry 'bout scum like us, see." The thought of cold, alcoholic drink turned Declan's mind to the bottle of strong Irish whisky under the pillow in his bunk, and suddenly he did not want to linger here chatting.

"Wheel, oi'm off. Oi'l see yers in de mornin', Taff."

"Yeah, and don't be late, boyo. I'll be looking for my own bunk by then."

"Don't worry yer little head, Taff. Oi can't wait to git back." Declan grinned broadly as he handed over the long-handled shovel.

THE SECOND DAY

Long before any of the passengers were awake, the ship was a hive of activity. The watch had changed regularly during the night, every seaman and officer taking his turn on duty. Bad tempered Breakfast Chefs crawled out of warm bunks, donned their whites, and went to join the Bakers, already hard at work in the kitchens. The cooking fires were lit and another day of strenuous labour started on the *Titanic*. Cabin Stewards began their morning rounds with tea, and coffee for the French and Americans on board, favouring those who they thought would produce the best tip for good, efficient service. The Dining Room Stewards began to lay up the tables for breakfast; the Barmen stocked their bars;   Cleaners attacked all the Public Rooms with buckets, mops and dusters;   Seamen swabbed the decks outside and polished up the paintwork and rails;   Stokers strained, with aching backs, to feed the hungry monster which drove on through the Atlantic calm, gobbling up the thousands of tons of coal in the process, in the only shipboard activity which was continuous as long as the voyage lasted. The temperature would not rise to yesterday's high, as the liner pushed on towards the Canadian Coast and the cold, ominous currents which flowed down from the Arctic Ocean.

The Captain appeared on the bridge earlier than usual: he was still a worried man. He rang down to the Engine-Room on the bridge telephone, keeping his voice low to avoid being overheard. He spoke to the Second Engineer.

"Everything alright down there... You know what I mean?"

"Yes sir," came the reply. "I checked Boiler Boom No 5 when I came on watch and it seems to be alright. I felt the bulkhead on the forward coal bunker and found no evidence of it heating up overnight. I don't think we need to worry, sir; I do believe the fire has burned itself out." The Captain would believe nothing without better evidence than a opinion.

"Just make sure nothing silly is done down there until we are sure, beyond a doubt.   I do not want that bunker opened, even for inspection purposes, until we reach New York. Is that understood?" The Captain waited for a reply.

"Aye aye sir."

"And you can pass it on to all concerned. The Chief assured me, and the Chairman, that we would reach our destination without having to touch that coal, and that is the way it stays, even if we have to burn your bunk when we run out of fuel for the boilers." The Engineer chuckled at the Captain's jest, but the Captain was deadly serious.

"Aye aye sir," the telephone repeated in the Captain's ear and he replaced the heavy instrument. Perhaps, because he had served much of his sea-time on wooden ships, where fire was the most feared of hazards, he might be over-reacting to this danger, but he was still not prepared to take any chances with over two thousand souls on board. The sea was a cruel element in which to have an accident, and a hard environment in which to survive after a disaster. Partially reassured, he turned to his proper duties, checking the ship's position, speed and course, and dealing with any problems which might have arisen overnight. This morning, there were none. Even so, he resolved to check Boiler Room No 5 for himself later in the day.

Continental Breakfast - croissants, rolls and toast, preserves, fruit and coffee - was available in the cabins but the ritual of English Breakfast was observed in the Dining Rooms, ranging, once again, from the solidly rural to the country-house-style depending on the status of the participants.

"Starting the day well" was a maxim at the time and all the means were available. Bacon with fried or scrambled eggs, boiled or poached eggs, kedgeree, kippers, devilled kidneys, sausages, mushrooms and fried bread were all on the menu; lashings of whatever was required, served on piping hot plates, with toast, freshly-baked rolls, yellow Cornish butter and marmalade to follow, washed down by hot beverages presented in silver pots to be poured into cups decorated with the White Star Line logo. The tablecloths were brilliantly white, crisp with starch, and would be whipped away for laundering as soon as the meal was over, whether they had been soiled or not, to keep up the conception of inviolate service and presentation. Standards may slip in later voyages but not on the maiden one, or the Chief Steward, with a pocketful of money already donated for expected effort, would want to know why.

Lorna Wainwright stayed in bed with toast and a refill of tea, which she did not really want, while Jonathan took the children to breakfast in the Dining-Room. It was not something he would have normally enjoyed but it gave him, at least, the chance to escape from the stuffy cabin for a bit, away from the cloying ambience of melancholy his wife's mood induced in the stateroom. He would take the girls for a turn around the deck after breakfast, he had informed Lorna, for if she was in the depths of despair, he, Claire and Alice must at least have some exercise and try to behave normally. He loved his daughters dearly, and even if the thought of trolling around the deck with their tiny, warm hands clutched in his was not what he was used to, it would give him a chance to look around and observe the ship's functions in daylight, if he could not examine such workings closely.

The trauma of the first day at sea was over, the excitement of experiencing something new beginning to wane, and the girls behaved very well in front of the American couple who shared their table. The woman had no children of her own, and was much impressed by the discipline of Jonathan's charges, despite their miserable performance of the previous evening; remembering the appalling behaviour of her relative's offspring, when they visited. Her enthusiasm for having children, at a later date, was quite restored.

"Is your wife not well?" she inquired, and Jonathan made up a story about Lorna being affected by the motion of the ship, this morning, to save a full explanation of her problems, which he did not care to discuss with complete strangers. Instead, he talked freely to his fellow passengers, wanting to know what it was like socially where he was bound, without realising, in typical English ignorance of other people's customs and tenets, how vast and diverse the United States was, and with such an international mix, that what might hold good in one place was not necessarily acceptable in another.

David Peacock retired to the gymnasium after a large breakfast. Molly made her way back to the Second Class to have her daily discussion with the nanny about the welfare of her children. David had dressed in a pair of white flannels and an old rugby shirt, sporting a large towel around his neck - he would go for a swim afterwards - apparently disdainful of the chilly air. He cut quite a figure in the company, and Molly's foolish doubts might have returned if she had followed him in there, for there were several young ladies present; anxious to trim expanding figures.

While he waited for his turn on the equipment, he struck up a conversation with John Sayer, an American travelling with his wife and son, with whom he had been on nodding terms in the Café Parisien on the previous evening.

"Devilish implements of torture, by the look of things, designed by some Torquemada, I've no doubt," commented David, eyeing the appliances.

"I have found during my time on earth, sir, pleasure invariably has its consequences, and the rectification of these pleasures always causes pain; cause and effect; self abuse requires penance. I'm a railroad man myself, travel in style too much: a good workout is long overdue in my case."

"Take my advice, 'slowly, slowly catchee monkey'," offered David.

"I'm not with you,"

"Don't overdo things; a little often is better than a lot all at once."

"I'll bear that in mind," commented Sayer, perceiving David to be some sort of an expert by his sporty dress.

The large, arched windows of the gymnasium let in a plethora of light, and the white painted walls and ceilings promoted a healthy atmosphere. Among the devices on offer were stationary bicycles, fixed to the wall, with a speed indicator in front of the masochists to help with accessing performance - this was the ladies' favourite although the long, cumbersome skirts they wore were not conducive to excellence of accomplishment - a rowing machine, mechanical horse and an electric camel. A map of the world hung on one wall next to a portrait of the ship, endowed with the legend "RMS Titanic. The largest ship in the world", on a wooden plaque underneath. The Gym instructor, T W McCawley, a powerful, stocky man, with obligatory clipped moustache and receding hairline, was on hand to give advice. David was soon ensconced on the rowing machine - he had done some rowing during a sojourn in academia - and was presently raising a good sweat and appetite for lunch.

The Chairman appeared on the bridge uninvited, just after breakfast time; safe in the knowledge no one would reproach him, because of his lofty position. He looked about, to see who was on watch, before he sought out the Captain and took him to one side.

"How are things going?" he inquired.

"As you see we are proceeding according to plan: all systems are functioning perfectly: the ship is in tip top order, sir," reported the Captain.

"Yes, yes, I know all that!" complained the Chairman - he had received a full report on the ship's disposition, from Thomas Andrews, over breakfast. He looked around conspiratorially to make sure no one was near before he said, "I am sure you know, to what I am allluding." The Captain coughed self-consciously.

"Yes, I believe I do," he declared.

"Well, man... ?" Really the old man could be quite difficult at times, even awkward when he wanted to be, the Chairman thought to himself, without realising how many of the Captain's toes he had trodden on the day before.

"According to the Chief Engineer, the bun... eh... our problem is contained at present. Several inspections during the night reveal the location in question is showing no signs of the fire: the bulkhead is not heating up as would be expected if complications had set in." The Captain tried to be as noncommittal as possible.

"Good, good. So it was all a storm in a teacup yesterday, I thought as much; not worth delaying the voyage over, eh!"

"I would not exactly say that, sir. One can never be too careful in these cases and a check must be kept on the situation until we reach New York."

"Quite! I am sure we are all in very good hands, Captain," In view of the circumstances, and the Captain's imminent retirement, the Chairman decided it was the right time to heal any breach which might have occurred because of his behaviour yesterday. "You know, I do not think I have ever told you this, but I have every confidence in you; always have had. Your departure from high command will be a great lost to the Line: we can always do with men of your experience and ability, and hope to find them to carry out our plans for the future which looks more and more bright. It is a great pity you have come to this time of life at the start of what will be the greatest revolution in marine development the world has ever seen! I wish we could retain your services for many years... but I know it is not possible." The Captain coughed again, in discomfort this time. He was not a man to indulge in soppy sentimentality, and did not take the Chairman's remarks as a deserving compliment; seeing them, rather, as the manifestation of an ulterior motive, whose purpose he would learn in due course.

"Yes... thank you," he muttered, and changed the subject hurriedly. "If you are at all concerned, I am about to embark on a tour of inspection of the ship, which will include Boiler-Room No 5, and you are quite welcome to accompany me," he offered.

"What, now?... I am afraid I have some commitments which preclude my immediate acceptance. However, I would like to come... I have not seen the ship in action, so to speak." The Chairman could have gone at that precise moment, but despite his temporary aberration in allowing his caustic regard for one of his employees to weaken, did not see why he should necessarily dance to the Captain's tune. "Look, I shall be free at eleven... Could you possibly delay your inspection until then?"

"Of course," agreed the Captain, "no one, except the ship, is going anywhere, sir."

"Good, good," concurred the Chairman in his annoying vocal style.

Lucas Meredith manipulated his overlong, slender fingers in front of the dressing-table mirror in his First Class stateroom. He liked to keep his hands supple: speed and control were essential when practising sleight of hand as any slip would invite disaster. He called himself a professional gambler, although his victims would not agree: they would come to regard him as a predatory cardsharp after they had been financially mauled by his lethal attentions. This trip had cost him a great deal of his carefully husbanded resources, and he needed to recoup his outlay very soon now or he could find himself in an embarrassing situation. Still, the means was at hand: he had arranged a game of cards for this afternoon, after a carefully planned visit to the Smoke-Room and the careful selection of his prey. It would start with a few hands of something innocuous, for small stakes - in which he would show acute recklessness and bad judgement - and proceed, hopefully, to a much more serious game with large amounts involved. No one he had yet come across could resist a sucker, in spite of whatever fortune they controlled, and Lucas, in his practised way, appeared to be the most noticeable of easy marks until he put his hands and brain into gear, and went in for the kill.

Lucas Meredith was not his real name, merely one of the aliases he used to ply his trade. He had been reduced to shipboard activities after he had been banned from most of the major Casinos in Europe when his ability to change odds, normally in favour of the owners, had been discovered. He did not start out as a cheat, employing a system of counting cards, and utilising a photographic memory, which had stood him in good stead when it came to making reasonable profits in his various enterprises. Denied a livelihood by greedy men who had to win all the time, he turned to finding lucrative card games but none of these lasted too long when his fellows began to suspect his talents. So he was finally forced to become a Card-Pirate, frequenting luxury liners, with rich passengers, and making a quick kill on the unwary, the innocent and the gullible. What he won before he was suspected would tide him over until his next booking - this class of person never welshed on their bets - and if he was uncovered for what he was, it would only be a few days before he was back in action on another ship. Of course, he would not be welcome where he had struck before, and although many ships plied the oceans of the world, the supply was not unlimited; hence his frequent change of name, and the necessity of having the documents to back up several identities, which all cost money to procure. He dreamed he would make enough money to retire one day, but he spent his winnings freely, and knew in his heart of hearts, he would never be free of the compulsion not only to gamble, but to take advantage of credulous men who pitted their wits against him out of greed. He was best at games in which the cards were not shuffled, counting being his forte, but had acquired other skills in card handling, along the way, for games in which they were. He was a passable Mechanic; a man who could manipulate the deal and end up with a pretty good idea what cards his opponents were holding. As a consequence, he did not lose very often, and on the whole, not much at all. Even so he had some ethics, and would not knowingly set out to fleece anyone who could not afford it, or go so far as to bring ruin or misery on any of his chosen targets; which was why he never jumped in feet first, and took his time with the selection process. The four victims he had picked out for his game today were all men of consequence, ruthless businessmen by the look of them, quite able to fend for themselves in a cruel world; all predatory enough to take advantage of their fellows; fatted geese just waiting to be plucked!

Lucas ran through his finger exercises yet again. He was a cool and calculating corsair preparing to go into battle; a condition he looked forward to immensely. Just pray that his luck held, and he did not run into anyone he had shaken down before, although it was not likely: his careful homework extended to checking the passenger list minutely. He regarded himself as an artist, not a malefactor, and the wealthy had a duty to patronise the arts, in whatever form they took.

Tom Pirbright did not have a good start to the day. Clara's sons, out of control through lack of their father's influence, behaved very badly at breakfast; squabbling, throwing food around and generally misbehaving themselves. For two pins Tom would have given them both a thick ear, but, Clara was very possessive and he did not want to start a family argument. They all had to live together for a bit, when they arrived in America, so he decided it was best to leave things alone. When the unruly conduct infected his own children, he did not stay his hand, and found himself in trouble with Amy: it was not justice, she objected, that some should be punished while others went excused. When the baby absorbed the mood and began to grizzle, Tom had had enough. He bolted his food down and made his excuses to get away; he could think of much better things to do.

He went in search of his erstwhile friends of the day before, mainly Dubliners and Liverpudlians, the live-wires on the ship, and found them in the Smoking Room. Unfortunately, they were not in the same easy frame of mind this morning, having over-indulged the previous night, and now nursing hangovers of varying degrees. There would be no tomfoolery for a while yet. He did glean from them there was going to be a shindig in the Open Space that night, organised by the leading lights, as no entertainment was laid on for the steerage passengers. Tom was urged to come, and he told them he would. Loath to go back to his cabin and face Amy, and the brood of children, he set off to explore more of the ship than he had seen so far.

His family was berthed in the bow of the ship, behind the crew's quarters, and as his natural high spirits resurfaced, he decided to be cheeky and see how far he could go through the ship, where he was not allowed, as he returned in that general direction. He would not get very far. He made his way to Saloon Deck D, via the Second Class staircase, and set off through the passageways lined by staterooms. It was all very posh here, he thought, much better than Third Class, with its cramped berthing and airlessness, the gift of the air-conditioning system which pumped out stale air to be consumed by the less fortunate passengers. One day, he decided, when he had made a fortune, he would return to England on this very ship, in one of these grand cabins, a glimpse of which he had been given through a door left open by a Cabin Steward. It was one of these stewards which halted his progress.

"Hey, what do you think you're doin', mate," a voice called out, and he found his way blocked by an effeminate man in a white mess jacket, the Cabin Steward's uniform. "You can't come through 'ere."

"Why not?" Tom challenged.

"Cos you're a steerage passenger, and you ain't allowed in 'ere," he was told.

"I got lorst," muttered Tom, "I'm tryin' to find me way up front, to vee... "

"Ooooh... trying to find the sharp end, are we, ducky?" cooed the steward, and Tom recoiled. "Well, you'll 'ave to go back, mate: you can't come through 'ere." The steward would certainly not have used this mode of address to his Second Class charges; Third Class passengers did not tip so he owed them no respect.

"Go on, mate, let me pass," pleaded Tom, trying to see more of the greener pastures, "save me va walk back, hey!"

"No," stated the steward obdurately, "you'll 'ave to go back, and that's that. Can't have my ladies and gentlemen exposed to the likes of you, now can we? Orf you go, mate, back to the lower decks like a good chap." The steward barred his progress, and the only way around him was through him, and Tom did not think it a very good idea.

"Fanks a bundle, mate," he declared sarcastically, and added, "When me shoes are worn aut, I'll come back and stuff 'em up your arse." The steward's face split into a broad grin.

"Ooooh, thanks very much, mate... I'll keep an eye out for you."

Tom was forced to retrace his steps. He had a good mind to report the steward to someone, but who would listen to him: the class lore which predominated on the ship decreed he should not have been where he was anyway: he would be considered to have been trying to rise above his station.

Leading Stoker Williams was completely exhausted when the Irishman arrived, ten minutes early, to relieve him. His slightly elevated position did not preclude him from hard work, but it had been some time since he had been required to put in a shift such as this.

"You're a sight for sore eyes, boyo," he enthused, "I'm long overdue for my bunk."

"If yers anything loike me, ye'll be dreamin' about dat shoovil for the nixt few hours," muttered Declan. The sweet redolence of stale alcohol slapped Taff across the face but he said nothing. The crew were not allowed to drink for the duration of the voyage - it was a sackable offence - but most of the stokers did partake from hidden supplies. It was a pretty hard life, down here in the depths of the ship, and these men toiled so hard, away from fresh air and light, they deserved a bit of comfort when off duty. Taff was Chapel himself, and did not drink, which was not to say he disapproved of others doing so in their own time, but woe betide any man, in his gang, who came on duty with a bottle hidden in his pocket.

"I think I'm a bit too tired to dream," complained Williams.

"Wheel, off ye go an' see," suggested Declan.

"Oh... I nearly forgot," Williams paused on his way out. "New orders from the bridge, boy, from the Captain himself, so the Second Engineer says... No one, not even Jesus Christ himself, is allowed to open the bulkhead door on the forrard coal bunker, see, or they'll cut off our balls and use them as bait to catch the fish for tonight's First Class passengers' dinner." He grinned at the embellishments he had added to the Second Engineer's orders: that should get through to anyone, even a 'dense paddy'. Declan grunted in reply: he had already suffered one niff of coal gas, there was no way he was considering opening the door to the forrard coal bunker.

Left to his own devices by the Leading Stoker's departure, Declan checked on his fiery mistress. Taff had done well; the fires, in the belly of the boiler, were well banked up. Declan felt a bit muzzy-headed this morning, and that was down to the amber whisky, contained in the bottle of Bushmills he had sipped from a little too freely last night. He had only intended to whet his whistle but had fallen foul of his old failing, the inability to leave off when he had the taste. He would run out before he reached New York, after last night, but had enough in his contingency fund to buy some more off a fellow stoker, to get him by, or bribe one of the off-duty stewards to get him a bottle from somewhere. It was a hard job getting the stuff aboard in the first place - the Master at Arms sometimes conducted spot body searches when the crew were embarking - and he normally managed his daily quota better than this. He could only put it down to the long hours he had been landed with: it sapped his strength and he needed to recuperate. As it was, he would have to make the return voyage with a bottle of American Bourbon for company, tough and palatable, but nowhere as good as the Irish Nectar. He shrugged. His condition was nothing that a few minutes hard graft, and the accompanying sweat, would not put right: he had done it all before, many times. He spat on his hands and went towards the rear coal bunker: it was a terrible grind having to cart the coal from this cache, which was going down fast, but it could not be helped considering the restriction placed on the forward bunker. Whatever would they do when the coal ran out? But then it was not his problem, only his place to do the drudgery when the time came.

Declan had not been shovelling for long when the little crocodile of men filed into the Boiler-Room. He recognised the Captain, the Chief and Second Engineers, but had never seen the man in well-cut civvies before. He did what he always did when officers were about, kept his head down and concentrated on his work, but his ears took in everything that transpired.

The Captain walked to the door of the forward coal bunker and put his ear to it. Whether he would have heard anything over the continuous hum of the rotating engines was debatable, but he seemed satisfied. He ran his hands over the door, and the bulkhead on either side, from the deck up as far as he could reach. The Chairman watched him intently.

"Well, it seems to be satisfactory," announced the Captain. "What do you think, Chief?"

"I don't think we have a problem, sir. I'm convinced the fire is out. We could open the door to see, of course, and if all is well, we could utilise the coal."

"No!" said the Captain adamantly. "I have given orders this bunker is not to be opened until we reach New York."

"I'm sure there is nothing to worry about, sir," persisted the Chief Engineer, "and we could do with the coal. The bunker aft is running a bit low: it is not going to last out."

"Then you will have to transfer coal from the other bunkers to eke it out."

"Is that really necessary?" cut in the Chairman, unable to keep out of the exchange. "It sounds counterproductive to me. We all seem to agree the fire is out."

"No," the Captain repeated huffily. "None of you present has my experience of ships. Fire is a devastating prospect while at sea. I think you should be guided by me... Sir." The Captain used the designation deliberately, trying to ram home his point, and Declan's ears pricked up immediately.

He stole a look. There was only one person on board the Captain was likely to call 'Sir', and that was a higher authority. So this was the mysterious Chairman that Taff Williams had mentioned, from whom orders emanated on high; the person responsible for all the extra effort which was required of him. He looked the Chairman up and down. The signs of good living showed in his puffy face, and in the way his frame, inclining to portliness, filled out his expensive suit. No, he would not be much use on a shovel, Declan decided, but he looked as if he might well benefit from the exercise. He caught the Second Engineer looking at him and dropped his eyes hurriedly: it would not do to attract the officer's attention: keeping a low profile was Declan's creed. He busied himself with his labours.

"Surely fire cannot be that bad in a metal lined compartment: there is nothing to burn except the coal." The Chairman could not help himself but interfere: he was a forceful character and had to be involved.

"We could stand by with a hose and..." began the Chief Engineer, but dried up when the realised the Captain was looking daggers at him.

"It is not the fire I am worried about: it is the time and effort, and the resources, we might need to employ which concern me. I am sure we all have much more important considerations at this moment."

"Yes, sir," mumbled the Chief, suitably admonished.

"Quite," agreed the Chairman, feeling responsible for the situation. The Captain turned on the Second Engineer.

"We have plenty of off-duty stokers, haven't we?"

"Yes, sir."

"Get a gang in, then and pinch a little coal from all the other bunkers. That will get us through," he ordered.

"But you gave orders no crew were allowed in here except Williams and Reilly," the Officer volunteered, turning his gaze on the Irishman. "What if the news leaks out? I mean..."

"They are only bloody stokers, man!" thundered the Captain. "You don't have to tell them anything: they don't control this ship: I do! Get them organised and put them to work." He turned on the Chairman and said very pointedly: "I hope that meets with your approval, sir!"

"Yes, yes," conceded the Chairman, "I am quite sure you know what you are doing." He put up his hands, palms outward, to placate the Captain, whose temper was visibly fraying at the edges.

"In this case, I do... Sir," snapped the Captain, and set off for other locations still to be inspected. The meek crocodile of men followed along in his wake.

When they had gone, Declan hawked and spat on the deck; the gesture a salve to his feelings of contempt towards his 'so called' betters. They had talked as if he was not here; as if he was insignificant; part of the fixtures and fittings; not worthy of consideration. If it were not for 'bloody stokers' like him, this great ship would not be hurrying on towards its destiny: for if he was only as insignificant as an ant, each lowly ant had his own value to the colony, and that, in itself, was deserving of some respect. They were so bloody snotty, the English, it was no wonder some of his people were in open, bloody revolt. Declan shook his head sadly at the injustice of it all. He had marked the Chairman well, in the few moments he had to examine the man: like Pandora's Box, all Declan's ills radiated from him. The Irishman would not forget his face.

The first ice warning was received in the Marconi Room about midday; it would be the first of many. Jack Phillips was on duty and he wrote down the complete message faithfully, checking the co-ordinates carefully. He sensed the importance of the bulletin - it was the first one which had been transmitted to him - and he realised it should be passed to the bridge at once. The wireless room was not very busy at the moment, so Phillips decided to take the cablegram form along himself. Harold Bride, the junior operator, was taking a nap, and Jack did not want to wake him. When such messages became routine, not so much care would be taken over delivering them.

Phillips arrived just as the ship's officers were gathering on the wing of the navigating bridge to calculate the ship's position in the traditional way, with sextants. 'Shooting the sun', as it was called, was good practice for all aspiring officers. Phillips handed the message to the Chief Officer and returned to his duties. The group of men moved into the chart-room to plot the *Titanic's* actual position, and work out the day's run. They had covered three hundred and eighty six miles in the first twenty-four hours: not bad considering they had left Belfast at one-thirty pm, the previous day, and the ship had not been run up to speed until she was well out into the Atlantic. The message warned of icebergs dead ahead, and when they calculated the position given, found it to be well to the west, in the Labrador Current. The ship was deemed to be in no immediate danger, and the Captain, still on his tour of inspection, was not informed at this stage. It would be two days before the liner would be close to the area, and a good look-out was maintained from the crows-nest at all times, in any case. The weather was fine and clear, visibility extending for several miles until the curve of the earth denied further perception. The officers returned to their duties and the ship sailed on.

Lucas Meredith flexed his fingers and began to shuffle the pack. Deliberately, he allowed several of the cards to slip through his grasp and fall on the green baize in front of him, as if he was clumsy.

"Oh dear," he muttered under his breath. The others watched him expectantly. He picked up the scattered cards and replaced them in the pack. "What shall it be, gentlemen? Rummy, whist, vingt-et-un... Oh dear, there are too many of us to play whist, aren't there?" he said, looking at his four companions.

"Blackjack," suggested John B Sayer, the Canadian Railroad man. It was the result Lucas was looking for, vingt-et-un by another name: the pack was not shuffled and he had every advantage. Considering the financial weight of his opponents, Lucas had decided to change his tactics this time. He would win a bit, as if with beginners' luck, and then lose heavily before becoming bored and suggesting his favourite game: poker. There was another Canadian in the company, Harry Poulson, of a Montreal banking and brewing family, and an

American, Manny Weidner, whose family fortune had come through building street cars. Only David Peacock was an enigma to Lucas: he did not say much about himself, but from the way he talked one could see he had been about a fair bit and seemed fairly well set up: capable of looking after himself; fair game! If he had known David was only here to make business contacts, and gain influence in the New World - it would be an advantage to go into meetings saying he was a friend of this magnate, and that - Lucas would have not entertained him at the table, because of his ethics. To gain credibility, Lucas hinted at connections with several English families of note - putting him solidly in the upper crust - making no mistake which could put him in the mire. He always did his homework very thoroughly before each voyage: there was nobody on board, whose kinship he claimed, who could possibly tip his hand.

Lucas could not fail to notice Sayer and Peacock had greeted each other warmly when they met. Sayer indicated the chair beside himself when he recognised the younger man, and they chatted like old friends while they waited for something to happen. This was why he had assessed David's status wrongly: he could have no way of knowing that because they had suffered pain together, in the gym this morning, a bond had developed, as it quickly does, when men share adversity.

"Who wants to be Dealer?" Lucas queried in a braying, false tone, sounding over-excited and rather foolish. "I'm not sure I can manage the Bank."

"We will cut for it, shall we gentlemen?" responded the serious voice of Harry Poulson, and they all agreed. Manny Weidner drew the high card, and began to shuffle the pack. It would only take a few hands for Lucas to get into the swing of things. Far from excited, a cold, calculating hand held his heart, and he began to watch the cards as they came out, and were returned to the bottom of the pack, in perfect concentration.

Lorna Wainwright quite literally bumped into Molly Peacock as she came out of her stateroom. The dark feelings which possessed her had turned to claustrophobia, and she had to escape from the cabin for a few moments. Jonathan was looking after the girls. Lorna had no idea where she would go, but she would not get far in any case. Molly had been waving good-bye to her children in the cabin next door, displaying childish exuberance, and she turned, after shutting the door, and started to walk away without looking. She walked straight into Lorna.

"Oh dear... I am sorry," she apologised as she stepped back, putting up her hand to straighten her feathered hat. "I was not looking where I was going," she explained further.

"It's alright. No harm done," Lorna assured her. Molly had to go on.

"I was visiting my children, you see, and I should have been paying attention... Are you the lady from the cabin next door? I do hope they have been behaving themselves and not bothering you. They are very good normally."

"I haven't heard a peep out of them," Lorna assured her. She was perplexed. "Did you say you have been... visiting them?"

"Yes. My husband and I are travelling First Class." When she realised how condescending it sounded, she hastened to confide, "Of course, we don't normally travel First Class, it's just that David... my husband... Well, his firm is paying for the trip, and we are treating it as a second honeymoon."

"How nice," commented Lorna. "Have you been married long?"

"Ten years. This year will see our tenth anniversary," Molly stated proudly.

Suddenly Lorna felt a lot better. Perhaps she had been doing wrong, locking herself away with her fears, missing out on the company of other females, to chat and gossip with.

"Oh, about the same time as us," she heard herself say. Then she giggled for the first time since coming aboard. "I'm afraid poor Jonathan hasn't an employer who would send us First Class."

"It is a bit of extravagance, I know, but I am enjoying every minute of it."

"Why not indeed? Make the most of it while you can has always been my motto."

"I am, I assure you, although I have not yet persuaded our Cabin Steward to find me some asses' milk for my bath." They both giggled together.

"I hear champagne is supposed to be a good substitute," counselled Lorna.

"I'm afraid my husband's firm might not go quite that far." They fell silent then, as they had run out of things to say. Lorna unexpectedly did not want to be alone; she did not want this refreshing woman to go away.

"Look, if it will be of any help to you, I could keep my eye on your children for you," she offered to keep the conversation going.

"Oh, that is most kind," crooned Molly. "They have Nanny with them, of course, but another pair of eyes is always beneficial."

"How many do you have?" Lorna wanted to know.

"Just the two. A boy and a girl."

"Ah... the same as us then, except ours are both girls." It seemed to Molly this woman had a haunted look about her, but there was something in her manner, something intangible, something desperate, which invoked Molly's interest.

"Is your husband going to America on business?" she inquired.

"Yes... well, no, not exactly. He is an academic, a Professor of Science... he is going to take up a Chair at a University," Lorna explained.

"My goodness," remarked Molly. "That rather puts my David in the shade. He is just a plain, ordinary business man by comparison."

"I'm sure he must be a good one if his firm is going to all this expense."

"Yes, he is: very good," confirmed Molly.

Once again they came to an impasse in the conversation, neither knowing what to say, or where to go next. Molly was the first to speak.

"It has been so interesting to meet you... I wonder... I have tea with my children every afternoon: I wonder if you would care to join us tomorrow... at four. You will bring your girls, won't you?"

"That would be very nice. I am sure they would enjoy it."

"I will arrange it with the Steward, then. Tea for six at four, in our cabin... unless your husband would like to join us?'"

"No, I think not. He is much happier with his scientific journals; not one for tea with the children I'm afraid."

"I did not really expect it. We will see you at four tomorrow, then."

"I will look forward to it," Lorna affirmed.

After Molly had gone, Lorna leant back against the wall of the passage. She felt much better now; no longer in need of a change of scene. What a difference a good chinwag had made, and she genuinely looked forward to the next day. Jonathan was a good old stick but not the brightest soul to be with; perhaps this mysterious lady she had just met could help to drag her out of despair. She went back into the stateroom a renewed person, and even Jonathan noticed the difference.

David had managed to keep up his end in the game of poker which followed the blackjack. He had not been lucky, never having much to go on, but he had confined his losses, surprisingly, to ten or twelve guineas. Chance had given him about one good hand in ten, but what he won had gone out in staking the next few games, so he was never seriously up or down. The game had never been that competitive throughout the session, just nice and friendly, with everyone winning a pot here and there, although Harry Poulson and young Weidner were the biggest losers by punting their money across the table, in trying to frighten the others out of the betting by raising the ante unwisely. The only one at the table who did not seem concerned whether he won or lost was the debonair Lucas Meredith, who studied his cards with a fixed, enigmatic smile on his handsome features; never showing emotion of any kind. He raked in his winnings without obvious glee, as was Manny Weidner's disagreeable habit, and accepted his loses with unspoken stoicism; the very model of a perfect gentleman.

It was John Sayer who broke up the game by pushing his chair away from the table.

"Well gentlemen, that's quite enough for me. I'll be gettin' it in the neck from the little woman for desertin' her so long," he announced unashamedly. Harry Poulson produced an ornate pocket watch and studied it for a moment.

"Me too," he concurred. "Besides, it's nearly time to dress for dinner."

"Good heavens," exclaimed David, "is it that time already?" Molly was likely to be in a mood over his long absence: they were supposed to be spending as much time together as possible, free of the children and the other constraints on their time occasioned by their routine in England.

"Doesn't time fly when you are enjoying yourself," observed Lucas Meredith. "May I suggest the same time and place tomorrow? I certainly would like another crack at you gentlemen; it has been a very interesting afternoon." A chorus of assent bubbled from around the table, although David was not sure he could make it. He really must consider Molly on this trip. "I'll be looking forward to it," said Lucas, and pushed back his chair to rise with the others. John Sayer delayed long enough to voice an invitation.

"You must join my wife and me for a drink after dinner. Shall we say the Palm Court at nine o'clock?"

"I'm sure my wife will be delighted. We have not made any friends on board. I should be pleased to accept."

"I'll see you later, then," David nodded convivially in reply. The Canadian Railroad must order their uniforms from somewhere, and what could be warmer in the Dominion's harsh winter climate, or harder wearing, than the Merino wool he had came here to sell? He could see a market opening up already.

David hurried through the ship to his cabin. He let himself into the stateroom, a hundred excuses to cover his long absence already formulating in his brain, to find Molly, stretched out on the bed, reading. She smiled sweetly when she saw her husband, which completely disarmed him.

"Did you enjoy your game, my love?" she asked.

"Yes, very much so," he confirmed. "I hope you did not mind my..."

"I met such a nice woman this afternoon," related Molly, cutting across her husband's lame apology. "She is in the cabin next door to the children: a professor's wife. Her husband is apparently on his way to take up an appointment in America. She seemed very sweet and offered to keep an eye on the children for me."

"Didn't you tell her we have Nanny doing that job," David reminded her.

"Well, yes: I mentioned Nanny of course, but she seemed so anxious to help I couldn't really refuse, could I? I've invited her to tea with the children tomorrow. She has two daughters of her own, and I thought we could have a nice little tea party."

"I hope you don't expect me to come," said David hurriedly.

"No, of course not, silly. I've no doubt the conversation will be about babies and things of that sort. We can't have you embarrassing... you know, I never thought to ask her name. Her husband won't be coming either; he sounds very stuffy, always burying his head in a book or magazine, by all accounts."

"Ah, I see," observed David with some joy, "all girls together, with lots of new gossip to debate." Perhaps he would be able to make it to the card-game after all!

"Yes, it should be fun. I haven't had a good gossip since... "

"Since the day before yesterday when you were at home with your cronies," David prompted, and she giggled.

"I've no doubt you will find some way to amuse yourself," she challenged.

"It so happens I have been invited back to cards at that time tomorrow."

"Well then, we will both be in our element."

David looked at his wife lovingly. It had been no mistake to marry her ten years before: he really had discovered a little gem.

"We are invited for drinks after dinner with a man I met today. I would like to encourage his acquaintance: I think he might be a useful business contact," he informed Molly, but she was not really interested. She had her mind on other matters.

"Just as you like, dear. You know, David, there was something quite strange about the woman I met today," she remarked.

"Strange... What do you mean strange?"

"I don't know really. It was not something I could put my finger on... as if she were preoccupied in some way. It is hard to say... just something strange."

"I've no doubt you will manage to winkle all her secrets out of her, dear, in your disarming way. I couldn't imagine anyone would be able to retain their mystery for long under your intense scrutiny," he said jokingly.

"Well, I am a woman after all," Molly replied.

Lucas was well pleased with himself. He had managed to control his avaricious nature: killing the golden goose before it had a chance to lay its promising bounty was not always a good idea. It depended entirely on the quality of the opposition. Gullible gamblers, with more money than sense, could be taken in one fell swoop, and there were two of those in his current selection, Poulson and Weidner, but the Canadian Railroad man played a canny hand and kept a watchful eye out for chicanery. Even so, the speed at which Lucas' hands could move would have deceived him, but it was best to bide his time while he set one of the others up for a big kill.

the casino, where his face, and his style of play, were too well known. Now was not the time for wishful thinking.

He had some time to kill before dinner was served - he was not subject to the inconvenience of having a woman to consider, and wait for, while she dressed herself in expensive finery: they had always been an unnecessary essential to him; games of chance being his overriding passion and providing enough comfort for his heart and soul - so he turned his attention to other things. He pulled an opened pack of cards out of his suit pocket and laid them on the dressing table in front of him. The cards were expensive and decorated on the back with the pennant of the White Star Line. No one had noticed when he picked them up after the game of poker had finished. Although a new pack, still in its cellophane wrapping, would be obtained from the steward before the game started tomorrow, the cards he had were still in good condition, and could be substituted at any time, after the new cards had been used for a while. No one would know the cards had been switched, so good was his prestidigitation, and all he needed to do was to set up his patsy hand. From his experience, and human nature being what it was, he guessed his fellow card players would probably take up the same positions as they had today: the herd instinct seldom failed to find a way out. He spread the cards out before him and went to work, concocting hands, working out cards for openers, what each man in the game would discard and draw to replace it, so four would stay in and one would drop out, until the betting became critical, when one by one the other two would fold, as they lost faith in the power of their hands, leaving him head to head with his victim. Just how far would his prey be prepared to go? That would be the excitement in the plan. He considered for a moment. Yes, Mr Peacock would go the whole hog; bet up to his limit and beyond: Lucas Meredith had seen his like before!

Satisfied, Lucas assembled the pack and tried out the deal, checking the hands to make sure it all came out correctly. It did. He set the sucker hand up to work out at David Peacock's position of today and then decided who would get what, when he dealt. John Sayer would be the one to drop out; keeping him out of contention, and away from harm; where he would not look too closely into the demise of the others. If he was wrong, Lucas told himself, and the players did not take up their previous positions, whoever got the target hand would be the unlucky one, although he had several other options.

If the man he feared, for his perspicacity, Sayer, was going to be the recipient, then he could stay the switch until another occasion, or, make his excuses to go to the toilet and put things right without chance of discovery. Glancing at his watch, Lucas found himself still with time to spare, so he ran through the deal several times. Despite the advantage his retentive memory gave him, familiarity with what he was doing had always been his maxim. He would continue to put the cards back into order and check the dispensing until he could arrange the cards in his sleep, to come out as he wanted. One little mistake could be disastrous, and turn his whole elaborate strategy back on himself.

Lucas had no compunction about what he planned to do or the means by which he would affect his coup. If these men were rich enough to travel First Class on the *Titanic*, then they were affluent enough to contribute to the Lucas Meredith Fund for a Continuing Lifestyle!

"C'mon gel," encouraged Tom. "It'll be a good knees-up! When them Irish blokes git goin', you can bet yer life it's gonna be a larf."

"Naw," returned Amy, "I don't feel like it." She was becoming more and more sluggish as she grew older, and the weight piled onto her small frame.

"C'mon, please gel. You'll enjoy it: ya really will," pleaded Tom. There was a time when she would dance all night, and the sight of bright lights, like those of a travelling fair, would send her into ecstasy.

"Naw. Who's gonna look arter the kids?"

"Clara," suggested Tom. "She ain't goin' nowhere an' she's got 'er own kids to look arter."

"I can't arst 'er. She's got enough on 'er plate as it is. Naw, she'll only moan if she has to look arter my three, and the baby ain't no joke to care for. It's about time ya realised that, Tom Pirbright."

"I'll arst 'er then," said Tom truculently. "She won't say naw to me."

"No you don't, Tom. I tole yer, I ain't goin' nowhere, an' that's that!"

"I'll go on me bleedin' own, then," complained Tom, slipping into the jacket of his cheap, ill-fitting suit.

"I don't know what's got into yer lately," retaliated Amy. "Vere was a time when you was quite content ta come 'ome from work and stay in all night with me and the kids."

"Don't yer see what we is startin' 'ere: a whole new life, gel; an exciting life? Vis ship is a wonerful place to be, an' I wanna be part of it! Having a bit o' fun, and a dance, and maybe a cuddle arterwards ain't a lot to arst, is it? Well, yer bleedin' well stay 'ere and look arter the kids, fur all I care! Vere was a time when yer used to be va life and soul of any place ya were at." Tom slammed out of the door.

"Tom! Tom!" Amy called after him plaintively, but he had gone.

Up in the Open Space the steerage passengers were letting their hair down with enthusiasm. Without the facility of a bar, they had brought their own supplies of drink, and bottles of bitter and dark stout washed down liberal swigs of gin and other spirits they had laid in to comfort themselves. Tom had no such supply but it was not long before his new found friends were sharing their generous hospitality with him. The Scousers he had latched onto were among the most vociferous present, fun-loving and full of high spirits: they would easily slide into the lower social strata of New York and Chicago, and become the back-bone of the growing communities in the years to come.

At twenty-five, Tom was approaching his prime, and was tall and well proportioned, now his body had filled out and lost its youthful gawkiness, although his features were too sharp to be called handsome. Yet in a uncultivated way he was attractive to women and had enjoyed many a sly appraisal, and not a few flagrant offers, when he did his carpentry work in houses occupied by frustrated women whose husbands were at work or away on business. Amy's increasing slothfulness annoyed him; it was not right she should stick to the children and deny herself the pleasures of life. She was two years younger than himself, and already beginning to look, and act, ten years older. It was not something he had bargained for, her mellowing and slowing down, when he needed an active partner as a foil for his vitality.

A makeshift band had set up at the bow end and were playing enthusiastically, if not quite together, as they struggled to come to terms with each other and the impromptu music. A violin lead the strains, with an accordion as the main accompaniment, while other less confident instruments tried to fit in down the line; Irish pipes with attached bellows; a penny whistle; an out-of-place kazoo. All in all it did not matter. The frenetic Gaelic rhythms infected everyone present and the excitement, as well as the beat, was transmitted to the deckhead by a hundred stamping feet. It was a far cry from the ship's carefully regulated orchestra in the reserved atmosphere of the Palm Court.

All about Tom, in the throng, the whining, nasal accent of the Liverpudlians dominated all conversation, and the good Irish names of their forebears flashed about from one to another; Mick, Pat, Sean, Seamus, Brendan and many others. Unconsciously, they were a mini-society that attracted most of the attention because they made the greatest noise. Although Tom's origins were from much farther south, in the tenements of the Capital, he felt at home here, in the bosom of his fellow countrymen; all tuned to the same thought; all elated and thrilled by the thought of starting a new life far away from the social obstructions of the British Isles, which would never let them rise to take, what they saw, as their proper place in the world - at least not in their lifetimes. In the New World they would each find their own level and for every mile the ship ventured nearer, the greater the elation.

It was then Tom saw her in the crowd. It was not that she was beautiful, just that she looked vibrantly alive, with flashing green eyes and flaming red hair, interested in everything happening about her, warm, passionate and with a ready smile: all the things Amy had been and no longer was. Unable to help himself, Tom pushed through the crowd until he reached her side. She took him in with an evaluating glance, and a genuine smile appeared on her full, red lips. She did not seen to be attached, and as far as Tom was concerned, it was in for a penny, in for a pound.

"Hallo," he greeted, "what's yer name then?" The girl was of indeterminate age, maybe as young as eighteen or as old as himself. She had gained the assuredness of womanhood and wore no ring of ownership upon her finger.

"Sian," she replied, holding him in the shine of her frank eyes, "if it's any business of yours."

"No, it ain't," he rejoined, "but I'd like it to be. D'ya fancy a dance?"

"Alright," she agreed and it really was as easy as that to pick her up.

A space had been cleared in front of the band and several couples were jigging about wantonly. Tom and Sian joined them, making an engaging twosome. It was not a dance Tom had ever done before, but the girl seemed to know what she was doing, so Tom followed her, too engrossed to worry if he was making a fool of himself with inept gyrations. It was some sort of Irish Reel they were engaged upon, requiring a rapid change of partners from time to time, as well as covering enormous areas of the dance floor in rapid motion, so they had no chance to speak. Tom tied himself up several times, missing his way, or the oncoming lady, as he only had eyes for Sian, following her stunning body at every turn, but nobody seemed to mind: good-naturedly pushing him back onto the right path when he erred in his steps. Sian was dressed in a long black skirt and a white blouse, despite the chill in the evening air, with only a plaid shawl to cover her upper body, as if she could handle the cold, or expected to be kept warm by the dancing, the crowd or perhaps, hopefully, something else. Tom could not but help himself; he was smitten and there was not a lot he could do about it. He hoped the music would end soon, so he could talk to her, but nobody had informed the musicians who ground on interminably, as if there was no real leader to terminate the melody at a given point, and it was the exhausted dancers themselves who ended the performance by drifting away from the improvised dance-floor. As they had been latecomers, Tom and Sian found themselves alone in the space, and stood there looking at each other while the band shuddered, uncomfortably, to a ragged halt. Sian was breathing hard, and the press of her bosom, against the white blouse, rose and fell rapidly; the fit, young Tom feeling no particular distress.

"You've never done that dance in your life," accused Sian, when she could make herself heard.

"No," agreed Tom, "but it were worf vee effort just to be whiff ya." Sian smiled again, cheekily.

"You luked like a monkey on a stick!" she chided, "I thought you could dance."

"Well, I can, but if ya 'ears monkey music, what d'ya expect?" he retorted, and they both laughed. "When vay plays a proper toon, we'll 'ave a proper dance," he informed her.

"Naa let's goan' find a drink, I could sup a bucketful arter that. Blimey, whiff all that goin' on, I fought I were a race'orse for a minute!" Sian took his arm and led him into the crowd. "Ead for me dah," she advised, "'e's gorra bottle or two."

Her parent was called Mick, and was already well into his cups. He was a big man, bigger than Tom, and florid faced; which could have been his natural colour under the carroty mop, or the result of his drinking. He greeted Tom with a mumble of words, but a heavy slur, and the unaccustomed twang, made him incoherent. Sian took a sip from a proffered gin-bottle and grimaced. She offered it to Tom but he shook his head in refusal: gin was a woman's drink as far as he was concerned. Sian searched the pockets of her father's heavy, poachers-coat and produced a pint bottle of dark stout: the glass stopper fixed into place with thick, shaped wire. It was more to Tom's taste.

"Where are you goin' in the New World?" Sian asked.

"New York," Tom told her.

"We are goin' to Chicago, like! Me uncle's got me dah a job in the stockyards there. They say it's the biggest yard in the world, like, and they're always in need of men."

"Where's yer ma? She whiff ya an all?"

"She died, like. There's only me an' me dah now. I could put in a good word wit my uncle, if you haven't gorra a job to go to." It was a direct invitation, and her eyes held out the promise of more than just a job offer.

"I've gotta job in New York," Tom muttered. "Me bruver an' me are goin' inta business."

"Oh well, I just thought maybe I could help, like... if you didn't have any wurk." Then she laughed. "We've still got several days of the voyage to go yet: maybe I can teach you to dance properly, like, before we arrive."

It was then Tom realised the impossibility of his situation. He desired this refreshing girl more than he had anyone since he first met Amy, five years ago, but what could he do about it? He had never even thought about it or realised he would get another chance. If he had been anywhere else - at home, in America, - he might have been able to get away with a double game, but not here, where people were packed in like peas in a pod. He had no chance of keeping his status secret: he could hardly pretend Amy was his sister, with no husband

and three kids in tow. Nor was there any hope of keeping Amy and Sian apart, because now they had met, Sian must surely notice Amy and the kids at mealtimes... unless... No it was no good, thought Tom, it was own-up time: he would have to come clean.

"Look, gel, I oughten ta 'ave started vis," he began awkwardly, the admission both saddening and sickening him. "I'm hitched, an' va old woman is 'ere, on board, naa," he added. It broke his heart to think she would go away, after his contrite confession, but Sian surprised him when she stood her ground.

"Why isn't she 'ere wit yer, like?" she challenged.

"She wouldn't come... She won't dance, an' that, naa she's got va kids. Me sister-in-law coulda looked arter vem, but she still wouldn't come. She ain't no fun any more," complained the crestfallen Tom.

"Well, if she can't be bothered to come, she won't be bothered if I borrow yer for a couple of dances, will she?" It was enthralling music to his ear.

Sian grabbed Tom by the elbow before he could reply, and led him back towards the dance-floor, where the band had struck up again.

"I'll teach yer to dance properly while I still gorra hold of yer," she warned. It was not a result Tom had expected after his candid admission but he was taken with the girl and wanted to stay with her.

Up in the Marconi Room, abaft the bridge, the messages for America were piling up. The Assistant Purser brought another batch about every two hours, but the *Titanic* was well out of wireless range of the eastern seaboard of the New World. Harold Bride was on duty, and he piled the message-forms on top of the growing heap. The ship would not be in contact with Cape Race, the most easterly station on the American mainland, until some time on Sunday.

Bride had given up trying to transmit messages through other ships for the time being: it was a lengthy business, time consuming, and a lot of the other ship's operators had closed down for the night. He had such a pile of forms now, it was becoming increasingly difficult to decide what was important and what was not. In any case, several of the other ship's operatives were turning unco-operative.

"Why should the passengers on the *Titanic* assume they owned the airwaves?" was the general consensus, and they put little blocks in the way to slow the flow; reception was not very good; their equipment was playing up.

The receiver began to burble and squeak, and Bride reached for a pencil and blank message-form automatically. He listened for a few seconds and then began to write. It was another ice warning coming in from the west, far ahead, and he wrote it all down. When the receiver quietened, he ripped the message off the pad and laid it to one side. Being a younger, less formal man than Jack Phillips, he was not overawed by his importance, or very interested in the functions of the ship. He would deliver the form to the bridge later, when he had finished his shift - if he remembered!

"What did you think of the Sayers?" inquired David.

"I thought they were nice enough," replied Molly.

They were strolling an the Promenade Deck, late in the evening. The night had turned very cold.

"I am hoping to gain some useful information from Mr Sayer... John," explained David. "He is the Vice President of the Canadian Grand Trunk Railway."

"Yes, as I heard several times, at great length, from his wife, dear," chided Molly. She shivered uncontrollably as a blast of cold air found a chink in the armour of her tightly fastened coat. "Why is it, the nearer we come to America, the colder it appears to get? If you look at a map of the world, our British Isles seem considerably nearer the North Pole than most of that continent, yet we are not afflicted by the raging blizzards, the low temperatures, and the terrible hardships of which your friend seemed so proud! How is that, David?" Molly wanted to know.

"I've no idea: I've never really thought about it," he admitted, both surprised and pleased by his wife's intelligent point. He really must try to spend more time with her in future: he had almost forgotten what a delight she could be.

"Why, my love: I thought you knew everything," she reproved jokingly, keeping the spirit of the evening going. David tried to recall the complexities of his boyhood geography.

"I suppose it is something to do with altitude. England is rather flat compared to the height of the Rocky Mountains which straddle the Americas. Then, of course, there are various ocean streams and currents to consider."

"Really," gurgled Molly playfully, "oh my, you are so clever." David laughed.

"I must own up! I cannot say why it is. Conceivably, we will find out during our visit to the United States."

Molly stopped and looked out of the large, square windows, on the side of the ship above the rail. Her mood changed.

"It does look so cold and dark down there," she commented. "I should not like to end up in the sea."

"Nor shall you, my love. Your adoring husband has taken the precaution of ensuring you are on the safest ship in the whole world." Molly was not convinced, it looked suddenly menacing, and she shuddered again as the icy fingers of the breeze reached out for her.

"Can we go down now: I really am quite frozen."

"Of course, my love," agreed David. He could think of many ways to warm her up, and one in particular stuck out in his mind.

"I must go," said Sian.

"Naw, stay a little longa, please gel. Va state ya dad's in, 'e won't miss ya till va morning," advocated Tom. "I'm enjoyin' talkin' to ya."

"That's not the reason I better go," Sian enlightened him. "You're a married man, like: yer should be tucked up in bed wit yer wife."

"Doan' be like vat, gel. She'll be asleep long since, snoring away like a pig!"

The crowd had drifted away as the hour got late, the drink took a grip, and the night became cold, until only they were left in the Open Space. No sign of life showed on the ship, except for the dark figures, behind the glass, keeping watch on the bridge. Sian and Tom stood in one of the shadowy corners, shunning the light: standing close together but not touching.

"Yer not very 'appy... wit her, are yer?" Sian asked.

"It's not fair! She used to be luverly, but ven ve kids came along an' she ain't va same any more," Tom divulged.

"Why do yer stay wit 'er, then?"

"What else is a man ta do?" replied Tom unhappily.

"Most men I know would luke for greener pastures, like," Sian told him.

"Well, yas, but I've got me job ta go ta: I can't let me bruver darn naa, can I?"

"Me uncle says there's plenty of wurk in Chicago. 'E says it's a looverly place, like. Besides, I'll be there," Sian reminded him.

"What's whiff ya, gel? We only met tanight," Tom wanted to know. Incredibly, she was propositioning him, and he was not sure whether to believe it or not. "Ya know I'm married," he grumbled.

"Any wife who doesn't luke after 'er man must be prepared to lose him," proffered Sian. "Anyhow, if yer ever in Chicago, like, luke up me dah in the stockyard: 'e'll know where I am. Now I must go." She started to move but Tom could not let her go. There was so much he did not understand: so much he had to find out about her, and himself. He grabbed her by the arm.

"Doan' go!" he pleaded. She examined him with her wilful eyes.

"And what do you want from me?" she inquired quietly.

"Ya know what I want. I jest doan' know 'aw ya feel abaut it," he declared. She reached out and took his hand in hers.

"Where could we go?" she invited.

"I dunno," he muttered lamely, wishing he had checked out the ship more thoroughly while he had the chance. The touch of her warm skin ignited his lust, and his knees began to tremble with excitement and anticipation. He could not conceive how this was happening to him, or why. He had no time to consider the ramifications.

"I'm sure we'll find somewhere," ventured the girl, and led the dumbfounded Tom towards the stairwell.

THE THIRD DAY

The good weather continued into Saturday, and the *Titanic* sailed on, untroubled, in a calm, flat sea. Even those passengers who were bad sailors had overcome the irksome effects of mal-de-mer on the smoothly running ship, which made no sudden turns or changes of speed to upset delicate stomachs. The dining rooms were full of hungry voyagers anxious to get value for money and the milieu rang to the sound of overworked cutlery and happy conversation.

Lorna Wainwright was a changed person at breakfast. She had enjoyed a good night's sleep, surprisingly, and the phantoms which had haunted her were fading away. She looked forward to this afternoon and the company of the woman she had met, briefly, in the corridor, outside her cabin. Jonathan was more than pleased when she announced, "I think I'll take a turn around the deck with the children after breakfast. You will accompany us, won't you, dear?"

"Of course," he replied, gratified to see her change of heart. Despite being on the ship with two thousand souls, he had felt lonely and wanted to share the little discoveries he had made on board, with someone. Now he would have the opportunity: Lorna usually showed some sort of interest in his recreation.

"I shall be taking tea with the women in the cabin next door, this afternoon," Lorna continued, then as women do, she began to elaborate. "Well, she's not actually the woman from next door: her children are staying in the cabin with their nanny. Her husband is a business man and his firm is..." Lorna went on, but Jonathan was not really listening. She seemed full of herself and completely back to normal this morning. He could only hope her dark fears would not return to cloud her mind. He did not like to see her depressed, especially by unreasonable concerns.

"Mmmm, dear," he mumbled when she had finished her short sermon, filled with his own concerns. "I hope you have not involved me in this tea party. You know how I dislike... "

"It is alright, dear, I have already excused you. You will have the afternoon to pour over your technical books."

"Ah... yes," he agreed, happy to be free, for a while, to go where he willed and do as he pleased. Perhaps this voyage would not be so onerous now Lorna had recovered her composure.

David Peacock looked forward to the routine he had established for the day. So many of his countrymen lived by the clock and he was no exception, initiating set patterns to keep his life orderly wherever he went and whatever he did. He would work out in the gym after breakfast, take a swim, have lunch, join his new found cronies for a game of cards, have dinner, and then visit the Cafés and join the society which frequented them. It was nice to have a regularised existence: it took the uncertainty out of life.

"I think, tonight, as a treat, we will have dinner in the à la carte Restaurant," he told Molly.

"Can we afford it?" Molly checked. "It does seem to be rather pretentious from what we saw the other day." David chuckled, it was Molly to a tee: always concerned about the little things in life, while the major issues, like political strife, and looming war, went straight over her head unnoticed.

"Of course we can, my sweet! What is money for if not to spend on the luxuries of life."

"This holiday in America is somewhat of an expense," she reminded him, "and might cost considerably more than we bargained for. I just wondered if it were wise to waste money on expensive dinners, when the fare in the dining-room seems adequate to me, and is already included in the price."

"I have taken the precaution of transferring enough money for our needs into a New York bank," he admonished her, although she would never have asked how much, or discussed explicit finances with him. "For once in our life we are going to have a good holiday, while we have the chance, so you will leave all the worrying about money to me. Tonight we will splash out! Dress in all your finery, my dear, and bedeck yourself with jewels, for we will rub shoulders with the titled this evening and I want to be proud of you as I know I shall."

Quite uncharacteristically, Molly leaned towards him and gave him a peck on the cheek - it was not really the done thing in these surroundings - but it pleased David.

"You shall be as proud as punch," she divulged.

"I am sure I shall," he agreed. They looked into each other's eyes and smiled warmly, consummately content in each other. Those around them sighed as they remembered their own youth, and understood, marking them down as a happy couple in the full enjoyment of their relationship: a sight, even here, to behold.

Tom Pirbright was not a happy man. He was painfully torn in two directions; guilt and devotion to his wife and children, and desire, now consummated, for the girl, Sian. Amy had stirred when he slipped into bed last night.

"Whassa time?" she mumbled.

"S'late. I bin talkin' ta some of va boys," he told her. "Go ta sleep naa."

"Ya've bin drinkin'," she grumbled. "Ya stink."

"Yas, some of va boys 'ad some bottles. Naa go ta sleep, will ya." He did not want her to wake fully, and hoped the smell of the drink hid the pungent smell of Sian's juices, which clung like a heady perfume; he could still feel the heat she had exuded. Even worse, he could not risk Amy waking and demanding her conjugal rights: he did not think he could have managed to accommodate her just then. Mercifully, she turned over and subsided into sleep, snoring fitfully within a few minutes: Tom need not have worried on that score.

For a long time Sian's image clouded his brain and he could not find oblivion for himself. What should he do now? Would this urgent feeling inside him eventually dry up and go away? Was this the proverbial shipboard romance; two young people overcome by the occasion; their destinies briefly entwined for a few moments in time; inevitably to drift apart when the ship docked and go on their own separate ways. In his case, Tom doubted that: he had tasted of the fruit and was lost forever. It was not something he looked for out of Amy's slothfulness; he had seen the girl across the room and the electricity between them had been generated; looking for a place to earth.

It had found a place, deep in the bowels of the ship. Sian had led him along forbidden corridors, deserted now in the slumbering liner. She tried every door which was obviously not a cabin, and found, at last, a Linen Room which some Steward had left unlocked. Inside it was warm and smelt of starched cotton with the pristine odour of newness still about it. There had been no long foreplay, just some passionate kissing, with wet lips pressed hard together, and fumbling hands exploring willing bodies. They discarded a minimum of clothing and meshed wildly, like animals. Tom, in his rampant excitement, was unable to sustain his driving into her for long; his spirit striving for blessed relief from the delicious ache she engendered. She clung to him ardently while he shuddered and thrashed to a climax, and then held him within her as if loathe to give him up. They whispered sweet nothings to each other while the passion subsided, but the girl encouraged his future interest by significant, wanton movements of her hips against him. After much too brief a time together, they adjusted their clothes, checked the corridor outside was empty, and stole away to their separate lives without making any arrangement for the next day.

Now Tom was burdened with remorse for what he had done, and how he had betrayed Amy. Yet at the same time he knew he could not give Sian up for as long as she was willing to receive him within her. It would be best if he made false promises, about what he would do in the future, and then take what advantage he could while the voyage endured, abandoning any notion of following her to Chicago, when the ship docked in New York. However, he already knew, in his heart of hearts, she would not be that easy to get out of his system. Then there was his future with his brother to consider, and Amy, and the kids. He loved the kids and his wife, but she had lost the carnal excitement Sian exuded, as she once had, and he came to realise this is what had attracted him to Amy in the first place. Now poor Amy's initial preoccupation with copulation had faded, and he had a responsive replacement, he was not sure what he would do, or how he would proceed from this point on. For so long now he had worked for, and anticipated, his future in America, and Bert would not be best pleased if he abandoned it to follow a skirt, but Sian was a beacon which would shine out to call him long after she had moved on with her father. And then, what of Amy, deserted and left with three kids to bring up in a strange land? She could not return to England as nothing had been left for her there: no hearth or home, no future without a husband to provide for her - and how long would Bert be willing to carry his brother's wife on his back while he struggled to salvage his business on his own? Yet, Tom knew, given half a chance, he would follow his heart, and his loins, to the end of the earth if he knew Sian was waiting for him there. It was not a problem he could resolve in a single, restless night. He must wait and see what tomorrow would provide. Perhaps Sian did not share his feelings, treating this as a casual encounter, but then that he could not ascertain until he saw her again.

He could not wait to get along to the Third Class Dining-Room, at breakfast time, for a sight of the redheaded spectre which haunted his dreams, and shouted at the children when they were tardy, hurrying Amy along when she made a languid effort to dress, until she complained, "Blimey, what's wrong whiff ya vis morning?"

"I'm 'ungry, gel, so git a move on, will ya."

"It's ya own bleedin' fault if ya's bin drinkin', ya's allus peculiar in va morning."

"Shaddup an' let's git on whiff it," he admonished, "I could eat a bleedin' orse." Thus he covered up his guilt by taking his frustration out an Amy.

All his haste availed him nothing: there was no sign of Sian when he reached the dining-room and claimed his table. Several other redheads peppered the throng, but none as bright as Sian, and he scrutinised each set of features without success. She had not turned up this morning, or had already been and gone; or had she been a dream, a figment of his imagination? No, he could still feel her sweetness engulfing him, as it had in the Linen-Room last night. Now in his disappointment, little things began to annoy him: Amy's and Clara's idle conversation, the children's constant bickering, the baby's small complaints. It all got too much for him: he had to know where Sian was, that she was alright. He pushed his chair out from the table and stood up, abandoning his half-eaten breakfast.

"I gotta git some fresh air," he announced.

"Blimey, a few minutes ago ya couldn't wait ta git 'ere cos ya said ya was I hungry," protested Amy.

"I phil sick," he reported.

"I dunno what ya was drinkin' whiff ya mates last night, but I'd lay orf it taday if I was ya."

"It ain't vat. I gotta queasy stomach, see; I fink I'm seasick."

"Yas, well, vey must be puttin' seasickness in a bottle ven," chortled Amy and Clara grinned at the jibe, in sympathy with her sister-in-law.

"Very funny," commented Tom dryly and fled from the dining-room. He began a thorough search of the steerage areas: he had to find Sian!

The Second Officer was taking a short cut through the ornate First Class Smoking Room when he spotted Lucas Meredith playing patience on at baize-covered card table, and he pulled up in mid stride. There was something familiar about the man, about the deft, economical way he handled the cards, but the officer could not put a name to him, or recall where he had seen the man before. He watched for a full minute, unobserved, as the card player was fully absorbed in his game, before he walked away. That was the trouble with this job: he had seen so many passengers in the course of his career, it was often difficult to put a name to a face: it could seem at times, as if every person on board had crossed his path before. However, something ominous stirred in his recollection at the sight of that face, and the feeling troubled him.

He sought out the Steward on duty.

"Do you know that man's name?" he asked, indicating the gambler.

"Yessir, 'e's Mr Meredith, sir." The name rang no great peal of bells in his brain, and yet the feeling, he had seen the elegant man before, persisted. He watched from afar, while racking his brain for an answer which would not come.

"Is there anything wrong, sir?" inquired the Steward, slightly pensive.

"No, I don't suppose, for a minute, there is," said the Second Officer, and strode away, leaving the Steward to stare after him. They were a funny lot, the officers, the Steward thought to himself; deep, as deep as Davy Jones's locker! There was nothing wrong with the nice Mr Meredith; he was an excellent tipper after considerate service.

Midday came and the officers gathered for the noon sight. The ritual was only forsaken if clouds obscured the sky, but the sun was clearly visible today, a bit weak and watery, but overhead, none the less. Some speculation broke out over the day's run when the position had been fixed, and a few small wagers laid, but the time for paying would not come until the fix had been transferred to the chart.

"Five hundred and nineteen miles, gentlemen," announced the Chief Officer when he had finished his calculations, carefully supervised by the other officers. "A good run! We are right on course and slightly ahead of schedule. The ship is making good time." He was pleased: if everything went well on the voyage, he hoped to succeed to the command when the Captain retired in a few days time, or at least to be considered as a replacement if another Captain was transferred to the flagship of the Line. No announcement had been made yet, but he had high hopes. He must try harder to promote himself when the Chairman was around.

The Fourth Officer was the closest to the day's tally of miles, and the others paid up reluctantly, not without some ribald complaint. The Chief Officer looked on benignly. He hoped to be these men's superior sooner that they realised, and their endorsement, in his new situation, would not go amiss: a new Captain needed his officer's support to smooth his path. Command was a lonely existence if discord reared its ugly head.

Tom was becoming distraught: he could find no sign of Sian on the ship where his presence was allowed. He cursed himself for a fool. If only he had taken her surname, or where she was berthed, instead of allowing his appetite for her to cloud his thinking, he would have been with her by now! His urgent questioning of others, in the crowd last night, produced only shrugged, negative replies. It was as if she had vanished from the ship overnight; lost overboard in the darkness. Much later in the morning he found Mick the father, in the Smoking Room, but the man was well hung-over from the previous night's drinking and was hardly capable of recognising Tom, let alone being able to say where his daughter was.

"I dunno: she's about somewhere," was all he would say. Tom, furious at the time wasted by the search, started to look for her all over again. Surely he would have to catch up with her sometime in their enclosed environment.

He abandoned the hunt at lunchtime - he was starving in reality by now and went to gather up his family for the meal. He got them all seated around the table, and sat down himself. He looked up and there she was, as large as life, across the room, where he could not go and talk to her, without raising Amy's suspicion. His frustration darkened into a foul mood. Disturbingly, Sian took no notice of him, concentrating on her meal, and Tom's continuous sidelong glances were entirely wasted: she never looked in his direction once. This caused Tom even more annoyance, and he had to desist when Amy started to seek the direction of his distracted gaze.

"Is vere anyfink wrong, Tom?" she inquired.

"Naw, of course not," he was forced to reply. He flicked his eyes in Sian's direction once again, but she was preoccupied. Tom decided he would never understand women, and their wiles, for as long as he lived. Thwarted, aggravated and upset he turned his fervent gaze away from the redheaded girl and tried to rivet his full attention on a lunch he no longer felt inclined to eat.

Sometime later, he glanced up and saw Sian heading straight towards him, and his heart fell. The determined look in her eye made him think some sort of confrontation, in front of his wife, was about to take place. He was wrong. At the last moment, when she was level with the table, Sian suddenly veered off her path and cannoned into his chair, sending it skidding across the polished deck. He ended up several feet away from the table, up against the back of another diner's chair. He leapt to his feet in alarm.

"Oooh, I'm sorry, duck!" apologised Sian, straight-faced, with the skill of an accomplished actress. "I shoulda bin luking where I was going." He dared to flash her a gentle smile.

"It's alright, luv: accidents 'appen," he told her. As she turned away, she returned his glance meaningfully, and hissed out of the corner of her mouth: "Open Space... tonight... after dinner," so no one else, but he, could hear. He nodded his head in reply almost imperceptibly, and then she had gone, out of the room.

"I wish some people would look where they're bleedin' well goin'," he moaned as he pushed his chair back to the table. Amy was quite unconcerned; already chatting to Clara as if the incident had not registered in her addled brain.

Congenial satisfaction swamped Tom's drained soul, and he suddenly felt hungry again. He attacked his food with relish. If Amy noticed another change of mood, she did not say anything.

David Peacock arrived in the First Class Smoking Room at precisely three pm. The other members of the card school were already gathered and seated at the table. He slid into the seat which had been left for him, next to John Sayer: the seat was the same as he had occupied yesterday. Young Weidner was on his right, with Poulson next to him and Lucas Meredith almost directly opposite. David nodded to his fellows. Meredith's face split into a broad, welcoming grin, as if he were the principal in the game, and the others broke into conversation animatedly, as if they had just been waiting for David to arrive.

"What a lovely day it has been!"

"Yes, and the ship seems to be making fine progress."

"I find the facilities so comfortable, don't you?" and so on: small talk designed to lower the barriers of distinction.

"Shall we carry on from where we left off yesterday, gentlemen. Draw poker? I don't think we want to bother with blackjack, do we? Not much of a challenge to the mind!" Lucas Meredith had taken charge. A new pack of cards, still in the fresh wrappings, reposed on the table in front of him. He had taken the liberty of purloining the cards he had used for his game of patience, this morning, and had a pack of cards in each side pocket of his jacket; both loaded to deal the patsy hand. He could deliver his coup de grace at any time he liked, as soon as the cards they would use matched the varying condition of either pack he held ready. The scenario was set.

A chorus of approval rippled around the table. Lucas stripped off the cellophane and took the cards out of the box. He hived off the jokers and returned then to the container. Very deliberately, he spread the cards out, face up, with a swipe of his hand across the table, so all could see: he did not want to give anyone the chance to say he had cheated by using a marked deck, which none of the decks he held in reserve were. He was not prepared to take any risks. When all had looked, he gathered up the cards and began to shuffle.

David took no interest in Meredith's antics, and used the time to look about him. To say the Smoking Room was opulent was an understatement. The club-chairs in which they sat were upholstered in leather, though brocade had been used on the arm chairs and sofas. The walls were lined with gleaming wood, stained and polished to an extravagant sheen. Electric chandeliers hung on the corniced ceilings, and linoleum tiles, with a square-scrolled pattern, graced the floor. The piece de resistance was undoubtedly the stained glass windows - one with a ship in full sail, and others depicting saintly figures which graced one wall, and mirrors had been placed in subtle places to make the room look bigger than it really was. The setting was a lot finer than any of the Clubs to which he belonged: a rich man's playground in which department, in this company, he was a fraud.

Meredith placed the shuffled pack in the centre of the table.

"Would you like to cut for deal, gentlemen? Highest deals: aces high." David cut and drew an ace. Perhaps it was an omen! The game commenced.

Exactly at four, Lorna knocked on the cabin next door. Her two girls were delightfully dressed in matching sailor suits; their long hair brushed into a torrent of flaxen lustre, which flowed down their backs to the waist. Lorna felt uplifted, unafraid now, at home even: about to rejoin the world.

Molly opened the door at her touch, as if she had been waiting just inside.

"Hallo again," she cooed. "How nice of you to come... Oh my! what pretty girls. It was very remiss of me yesterday, not to introduce myself. I'm Molly Peacock."

"Lorna Wainwright, and these are my girls, Claire and Alice."

"How nice to meet you," uttered Molly as she stepped aside to usher her guests into the stateroom. Her own children were much of an age, and the introductions were made. "This is John, and Rebecca... and we mustn't forget Nanny, of course." Nanny was a grizzled old maid in her late fifties - she had been with the family a long time: David was among her previous charges - and of stern countenance; unbending in her approach to discipline. In all respects she was a treasure: she loved and cared for her wards with a concern which could not be equalled, and she knew, and fitted into, her place. She immediately took charge of the children and led them away to a discreet distance, leaving the two women to sit down and enjoy the freedom of uninterrupted conversation.

"It is so good of you to come," began Molly, "I haven't really had the opportunity for a good chinwag since we came aboard. My David keeps introducing me to the wives of the people he meets, and hopes to do business with in America, and although I have to be pleasant, he does not seem to understand they are either not of equable age, or my particular cup of tea. I do not find I have much to say to them."

"I am afraid I have not made any friends. Jonathan is not one for socialising outside his academic set, so we have stuck pretty much to our cabin." Lorna told a white lie to cover her own inadequacies.

"Oh, how unfortunate for you, dear," commiserated Molly, and Lorna hastened to set the record straight.

"It is not that he is unsociable, you understand. It is just that his mind does not work on the same plane as us other mortals, and he needs more than ordinary conversation to stimulate his mind. If small talk is not about the marvels of the age, he finds it very boring."

"I quite understand. We seem to have found ourselves very different types of husband. My David constantly talks to all and sundry, to see what advantage he might gain, and I sometimes wish he could be more circumspect and discerning, as your husband appears to be," stated Molly.

"For my part, I wish I might borrow your husband from time to time, as it can be very boring to have matters discussed with you constantly, which quite frankly, go right over my head most of the time. I am afraid that is the price you have to pay for life with an academic. It would be quite refreshing to escape to the normal world now and again." Molly giggled.

"Perhaps we could arrange to exchange for a while, sometime in the future."

She regretted the remark the moment it had popped out of her mouth, in case Lorna misunderstood her humour, and took umbrage. She had underestimated her guest. Lorna giggled too.

"Perhaps, it would make a nice change for us both," she agreed.

A short silence followed as both women considered the implications of what had been mooted. No spouse is ever totally satisfied with a partner, but the conversation was never intended to be serious. Molly was not one to let things fizzle out at that point.

"Where are you from, Lorna, dear?"

"Oxford."

"Oxford!" echoed Molly, "My brother-in-law, Jack de Vere, attended Oxford. He married David's youngest sister, Gladys, and took her off to Central Africa," she confided as if Lorna was a family friend, catching up on the news. "It must be a terrible hardship to have to uproot yourself and move to America. We are only going for a holiday, after David has concluded his business."

"Yes," agreed Lorna. "I did not want to leave England, I must admit. But then Jonathan decided his future is in the United States. He has taken this University Chair as a stopgap. When the opportunity arises, he will move into industry, into research if he can find the funding. He says recent innovations, like the use of electricity, and the invention of wireless, will open up a whole new field of possible discoveries which will change the world forever. When he has found the right sphere to concentrate his efforts on, he will return to England. American entrepreneurial skills coupled with British craftsmanship should produce commodities which will be the envy of the world, he has decided, so I cannot return to my little home in Oxford until he has learned them." Lorna broke off as if in distress. "One must be supportive of one's husband," she added wistfully.

"Quite so," offered Molly, "although I am not sure I could give up my beautiful home for such a venture."

"Oh, it is not that our house is anything grand - Jonathan is far from affluent - but it is the sentimentality which draws me to home: we have lived there since first we married. On well, I suppose it will still be there when I return." So this is what she had sensed when she first met Lorna, Molly decided; a deep melancholia over being moved away from the place she loved to the other side of the world. Molly was glad she had thought to invite the woman to tea. Perhaps it would not be so bad for her if she had a shoulder to cry on! Even so, Molly pondered on the unfairness of life. Here was David, academically disadvantaged compared to Jonathan, yet making good money because he was a successful businessman, and the poor Jonathan, undoubtedly brilliant by the sound of it, having to displace his family, and go to America, in order to open up options for his future.

"Did your... David... attend University?" Lorna inquired.

"No, he went straight into the family firm after he left Public School." Molly had to own up. She felt like a fake as it was, travelling in First Class, and could not try to put herself above her new found friend, especially one who had renounced so much in support of her husband. "It is not our family firm, actually," she divulged, "it is the de Vere Wool Company he works for. David's family have lived next door to the de Veres, in Forest Hill, for over a hundred years, and are intermarried and closely associated. The de Veres are of lofty stock, claiming descent from the Normans who came over with William the Conqueror, but make very bad businessmen. They are soldiers, highly-placed clergymen and statesmen, not given to the intricacies of commerce, in which David's relatives excel, so it is an equitable arrangement which works to the advantage of both families."

"How interesting to have such a lineage!" commented Lorna, not sure how she should respond. Molly continued unabated.

"David has done so well in the firm, he is Director in charge of procuring new markets, which is why we are travelling to America: he has great hopes for trade there. Normally he travels the world in search of business, and I am left at home to stagnate until he decides to reappear."

"How exciting!" enthused Lorna, and then checked herself. "Well, for him at least. It must be terrible for you to have to sit and wait for his return from these foreign trips."

"Yes, it is," concurred Molly soulfully, "but then, I, like you, must support my husband, so as not to cramp his ambitions." The conversation was terminated by the arrival of the Cabin Steward with afternoon tea, but a bond of sympathy, for each other's plight, had been forged between the two women.

It was a traditional English tea that Molly had ordered. Thin cucumber sandwiches adorned the plates, along with an assortment of cakes, scones, and biscuits. The tea itself, and hot water, milk and sugar, were served in silver pots and bowls, all engraved with the Company crest. The tea-plates, cups and saucers were marked with the blue motif beneath the glaze: no expense had been spared n the *Titanic's* outfitting. The children were served first, helped to plates of goodies, and then banished to the periphery of the stateroom, once more, under the eagle-eye of Nanny, who would not let their elders be bothered by them. They were getting on quite well, the children; brought up to the same standard of upper middle class behaviour by adults obsessed with ensuring they fitted into the right niche that society was reserving for them. However, they could not have been more different: the Wainwrights, blonde and pale skinned, the Peacocks, ruddy complexioned and copper-headed, influenced by their father's dominant genes.

"You know, Molly," Lorna revealed, "I am so pleased I took up your invitation. I must confess, when I set foot on this vessel, I was overcome with the feeling some disaster would overtake us, and very depressed by it."

"But that is absurd," protested Molly. "David says this is the safest ship afloat. Whatever could have given you such an idea?"

"I don't know, it is just a terrible foreboding which came over me." Lorna felt a lot better now she had confessed her fears to this supportive woman. "Jonathan told me I was being very silly, but I could not shake off the feeling until I met you. Now it seems only an unpleasant memory... I shall be eternally grateful to you."

"Nonsense, dear," objected the practical Molly. "You, like me, were depressed because you had not engaged in a good gossip for so long!" Both women chuckled conspiratorially.

David was becoming bored. For the second day running, his luck had been sporadic, and if it did not change, very soon, to the good, he would abandon this game and find other distractions for the rest of the voyage. Hand after hand was weak, and what he drew from the pack was always near to filling up his hand, but never good enough. His acquaintance, John Sayer, had endured much the same as himself, winning only the odd hand, and staying just about level in money. All the action had happened on the other side of the table, with Weidner and Poulson punting recklessly, and the solid Meredith accumulating steadily, much the same as yesterday. David struggled to remember the last time a hand occurred when more than two of the players had been prepared to bet: perhaps it would have been better to strip the deck down to a lesser number of cards, to make it more interesting, instead of using the full pack. To relieve his flagging interest, he might even suggest it, if the next few hands proved as unproductive. He had not came here to win vast sums, but a little reward for his efforts would not go amiss.

He pulled a cigar from the leather case beside him, on the table, and snipped the end with the gold cutter, from his waistcoat pocket, which had been one of Molly's birthday presents to him. He lit the cigar with a match and blew a plume of smoke towards the ceiling. Having just thrown in a useless hand, his heart was not in the game, so his attention wandered. The signs were not unfamiliar to Lucas Meredith, and he knew the time to strike was nigh. David watched the Steward delivering a drink, a brandy by the look of the dark spirit, on a silver tray, to a well-set-up gentleman, ensconced in an armchair nearby. He licked his lips, as he imagined the taste of good brandy trickling between them and assaulting his throat: perhaps he would be better employed in the bar. He speculated on whom the gentleman might be, and whether he might be some sort of useful contact in the New World.

It was Meredith's turn to deal and David did not bother to watch him as he prepared to deliver the cards. At the last moment, as his fingers were about to move, Lucas was suddenly engulfed by a disturbing coughing fit, which racked his body, and threatened to dislodge him from his chair. He turned his body away from the table, apparently doing the gentlemanly thing by not expectorating over his companions, and rode out the spasm until he recovered. Breathing in and out, deeply, he turned back to face the table. The pack lay undisturbed in his left hand.

"Excuse me, gentlemen," he apologised, then fixed an accusing stare on David, across the table from him. "The fumes from your cigar, I believe, sir," he remarked. "I am not a smoker myself!"

"I will keep my 'fumes' to myself, in that case," retorted David, having no intention of stubbing out his cigar: it was the only bit of pleasure he was getting from this dreary afternoon. Lucas switched off his indicting glare and began to deal. No one objected. Nobody had observed the cunning switch.

David picked up his hand, idly, and looked at the cards. He had two aces, a jack, a seven and a five: enough to open with. It caused no great stir in his mind: he had been dealt several similar hands which had come to nothing. What should he do? He decided to hold the aces and jack, in case two pairs, or better, a full-house, might come up, but the odds on that were very long.

"Anyone open?" inquired Lucas. Harry Poulson studied his hand and then passed. Manny Weidner followed suit. David was disinclined to open - his hand was certainly strong enough, but then, if the others passed too, he would miss the chance of a small pot.

"I'll open," he announced, and threw a guinea into the centre of the table. All the others paid to join him.

"Cards, gentlemen?" ventured Meredith. David watched to see what the others would do. Poulson took two; Weidner three; two for himself; John Sayer demanded four; Lucas Meredith took three. David was the last to lift his cards from the green baize, and stared in disbelief, trying not to let the emotion show on his bland face as the adrenaline pumped through his veins at the sight. He had drawn another two aces, and sat with all four in his hand. In all the years he had played this game, in the good times and bad, in many parts of the globe, he had never seen all four come out together: it was a million-to-one chance. He had seen, and held, four-of-a-kind many times, of course, but never all aces, and did not think he could be beaten by anyone around this table! "Well?" asked Meredith, from across the table, and David, trying to disguise the faint shake in his fingers by scratching the side of his nose with his spare hand, failed to notice the predatory look in the cold eyes which watched him closely, never deviating for a second.

"I will go a guinea," said David quietly, and threw another coin into the pot.

John Sayer looked at his hand. He had been delivered the usual rubbish, and retained a king to see what he could pick up. Nothing came and all his cards were different, except two which were of the same suit. He threw in his hand disgustedly.

"Carry on without me," he said. Meredith pushed his money into the centre without taking his eyes off David. Harry Poulson had retained a five and six of hearts, with a seven of clubs. He drew an eight of spades and a four of clubs. He had a straight. It was the best hand he had picked up for sometime, and he put his bet in. Manny Weidner thought it was his birthday. He had held a queen and a ten, and picked up two more queens and another ten to fill up his full house. He staked his money a little too hurriedly, raising the bet to five guineas. David complied, then Meredith and Poulson. Weidner raised the ante to ten and the others followed suit, and then went around again, none of them prepared to pack their hands in at this stage.

It was Lucas Meredith who broke the pattern.

"We all seem to be holding good cards. Shall we make things more interesting. I will bet fifty guineas I have the best hand of the lot." Poulson followed without hesitation, and Weidner followed him. David checked. The betting was getting out of hand and he was running short of money on his person, yet he could hardy stop the game while he went running to the Purser to change a cheque. He studied his hand. There was no way he could lose with four aces: only a running flush could beat him. He remembered what cards the others had drawn; Meredith, three; Poulson, two; Weidner three. What man would have the luck to draw three, or even two cards, of the right denomination and suit, to fill up a running flush: the odds against that were enormous, incalculable. If any of them had held four cards and drawn one, he would have worried, but the best that could be ranged against him was a full-house, a flush or a run; more likely three-of-a-kind or two high pairs. He could not lose with the hand he held. It made up his mind for him.

He looked up to see Meredith's eyes locked onto him, half open under heavy lids, like a Gila Monster sunning itself, yet deadly, and always ready to pounce with its fatal, unshakeable bite set in a hideous grin. David still failed to recognise the signs; he considered this to be a friendly game.

The challenge from the faces across the table was unmistakable: they were anxious to get on with the game.

"Excuse me, if I delay, gentlemen," said David, "but I am running short of cash. If I am to continue in the hand, you must be prepared to accept my marker. If I lose, I will settle my losses with a cheque. Is that acceptable?"

"We are all gentlemen here, are we not?" observed Poulson. "Surely we would accept each others' markers?" Weidner readily agreed. Only Meredith delayed his answer. It was not quite what he had expected: cheques could be stopped at a later date, and were always suspect, but then he had no reason to believe Mr Peacock was not a gentleman, and as true as his word. It would have to be off the ship and into the bank with his prize, at the earliest opportunity, when they reached New York, plus the necessary expense of a special clearance. Nor had he reason to suspect his victim was not a wealthy man.

"It is fine by me," he agreed. David raised the bet to a hundred guineas, and the first of his markers, from the pad he carried in his wallet, was placed in the pot. The notes began to pour in as the gold coins ran out and still none of the four men would yield, until Poulson cracked, doubting the strength of his hand in this company, yet fearful in case he lost out.

"This seems to be getting out of hand. This is a friendly game, isn't it? Shall we all turn our cards over and let the winner take all," he suggested.

"On no account," objected Meredith, even knowing he could not lose. He had not finished yet, and only a quarter of the profits he expected to take sat on the green baize. "We shall play the hand out," he insisted.

"In that case," abjured Poulson, "you can count me out. This is a little too rich for my thin blood." Once again David wondered if he was being wise, but his confidence returned when he looked at the pile of money in front of him.

It was an excellent bonus to pick up, and would more than cover the cost of his projected holiday, with Molly and the children, in America.

"As our friend previously stated, we do not seem to be getting very far with this," Lucas said deliberately, when it was his turn. "With your permission, and as no limits were mentioned, I am going to raise the bet to five hundred guineas - that should sort out the men from the boys, eh what!" He was braying again, trying to evoke a picture of irresponsibility. John Sayer sucked in a draught of breath as he heard the proposal, and it helped to put an end to the short, sanguine reverie David had allowed himself. Sayer was staring at him hard, as if willing him to discard his hand, but David was confident he would beat them all.

"It is alright by me," he heard himself say, and Meredith smiled in satisfaction.

"Of course, cashflow being what it is, I shall have to present my own markers," he checked.

"Of course!" David inclined his head slightly in deference. Weidner was considering his hand now, beginning to doubt the strength of his full house.

"I'll go," he decided at length, and reached out to drop another thick wad of notes onto the table.

"I will go once more to test the temperature of the water," said David decisively, and scribbled another note on his pad. Meredith too wrote out a chitty for five hundred guineas and placed it in the pot without saying a word.

Manny Weidner looked at his hand again. He was getting close to the limit of his allowance, and had to decide whether he should forgo his pleasures, for the rest of the month, on the off chance of winning the handsome pot. It was not an idea which appealed to him.

"Go on," he muttered dejectedly, dropping his hand onto the table in front of him. David looked into Meredith's cold eyes, trying to read what the man might be holding. He saw nothing in them which gave him any clue.

"I shall go again," he said coldly, reaching for his pen.

"And me," countered Meredith, a little too hurriedly, doing likewise. The first sound of warning bells rang in David's brain: the man was a little too cocksure. What on earth did he hold? It had to be another four-of-a-kind for him to be so confident, in which case David had the beating of him: nothing ranked higher than aces. And yet, there was something about the man's contentious demeanour which frightened him, almost as if Meredith knew he could not be beaten; but how could that be?

"As this is a friendly game, and to limit any further financial damage which might lead to acrimony, I shall have to see what you have, for a further five hundred guineas," David uttered between almost clenched teeth. The tension between the two men crackled in the stilted atmosphere.

"As you like," shrugged Lucas, having achieved his coup. Yet he waited while David wrote out another marker, watching him until he had placed it in the piled-up kitty. David returned the top to his pen and placed it in his jacket pocket. He could hardly watch as Meredith faced his cards one by one.

Lucas turned over the two of diamonds, then the three, the four, the five and the six.

"Low straight," he announced, "all of the same colour," and looked across at David expectantly. John Sayer let out a mammoth sigh and the hammer of despair crushed David's spirit.

"Beats me," he mumbled despondently, and dropped his cards onto the table in front of him.

"What did ya have? What did ya have?" demanded Manny, trying to scrabble up the jettisoned hand, but David knocked his arm away roughly, and placed his cards in the centre of the pack where no one could see them.

"That, sir, is my business!" he said angrily, half turning on the youngster, his eyes blazing, and Weidner cowed away, as if expecting to be punched.

"Anyone for any more?" queried Lucas quite cheerfully, gathering in his winnings. He began to count out David's markers, placing them in a pile.

"No, I do believe I have had enough," muttered a distraught David.

"You look like you could do with a drink," suggested Sayer, as the enormity of what had happened began to register on the younger man's face.

"I make that two thousand, four hundred pounds, give or take a few guineas, but I'm sure we are not going to argue over that!" Lucas held out the chits to David; the challenge blatant in his eyes. "Would you like to check?"

"No," snapped David, under the considerable pressure of what he had to face.

"And when can I expect your cheque?" Lucas asked cheekily, putting the boot in with both feet.

"This very instant," stormed David, fumbling in his pocket.

"That would be most acceptable. The name is Meredith, Lucas Meredith, that is with two 'e's' and one 'i', if you please." This afternoon's work had given him a great deal of satisfaction. Then the mocking tone disappeared from his voice, his victory won, and he became conciliatory. "I say, bad luck, old chap, but it was a rare old contest, what! In normal circumstances, I would want to keep the winning cards after a hand like that, but I think you deserve them as a souvenir." He collected up all the cards and handed the pack to David in exchange for the cheque, which he stuffed into the breast pocket of his waistcoat briskly, noting with satisfaction, that David put them, almost absentmindedly, into his coat pocket. It was the nucleus of Lucas' plan, should any inquiry be forthcoming, that the cards were available to be examined, and then anyone would be able to see they had not been tampered with. The effect would not be the same if he produced the pack, if they already doubted his honesty, and then no one could disprove that Lucas Meredith was not a extraordinarily lucky men, or talented in the execution of his given trade.

Molly had been waiting for sometime when David let himself into the stateroom. She was wearing her best evening gown, a shimmering blue, with her black hair neatly coiffured, and the merest suggestion of make-up on her face. She looked very pretty, delightful. A solitary diamond sparked from the pendant at her throat, and several rings flashed, on her fingers, as she moved her hands up to cover her cleavage. Despite the delay in his arrival, David's sudden entrance had startled her. His eyes were strangely wide open, wild looking, and the expression on his face was black as thunder; not a pleasant sight to behold.

"David, where have you been? It is almost time to leave for the Restaurant and you are not even dressed yet," she railed at him.

"We will not to going to the Restaurant... not tonight," he told her: his tone gravely aggressive.

"But you said we would," she complained. "I've gone to the trouble of getting ready in my best clothes."

"You were right," he informed her. "We cannot afford it... not now." David came closer. He staggered slightly as he walked and he stank of fresh, raw liquor. Molly's spirits sank, as the lovely mood she had been in, after this pleasant afternoon, evaporated. She had never seen her husband like this before, and her skin turned ashen beneath the slightly pink powder she had applied to her face.

"David! What ever is the matter?"

His shoulders slumped as the aggression drained out of him, and he came close to her, like a small boy brimming with contrition.

"I'm sorry, m'dear. I have been rather foolish... acted unwisely. No, I've been a bloody fool. I have lost all my money in a card game," he confessed, and at that moment it did not seem so bad to Molly. She had never been short of money in her life, coming from a rich background, and her husband had always provided for all her needs. Having no money was a situation of which she had no understanding.

"You mean all the money you had on you?" she verified. "Surely that is no great problem? Why don't you change a cheque with the purser?"

"You do not understand!" wailed David. "I said 'all my money'. I meant all the money I transferred to America and more. I shall be hard put to meet my obligations." Molly was dumbfounded.

"How much did you lose?" she breathed.

"Over two thousand pounds," he owned up unhappily, and Molly gasped. It sounded like an enormous amount of money to her.

"What possessed you to do that?" she demanded.

"It was the most incredible bad luck. I had a hand that could not be beaten and yet it was."

"How could that be? It could either be beaten or it could not be beaten." Her practicality reared its head again.

"You don't understand. I meant it should not have been beaten in a million years, but someone had a higher hand." Molly was not concerned with ambiguous trivialities.

"What does this mean?" she snapped.

"It means we have no money. I transferred all I had in my account to America; two thousand pounds, so we could have a good holiday. You know I am paid annually. I have only just been paid."

"You mean we will have no holiday now?" she asked as her bottom lip began to quiver. "Oh David! I was so looking forward to it! And the children... they will be so disappointed."

"No," he confirmed. "There will be no American holiday. I have my expenses to come from this trip, of course, but it will not be enough to last us a year at the rate we live. I will have to sell some shares and borrow to cover my liabilities, I'm afraid. I can hardly go cap in hand to old de Vere, and ask for an advance on next year. We will have to return home as soon as my business is concluded. I am so sorry, my dear."

"How could you do this?" Molly demanded, and David's features crumpled under the strain he had been forced to bear. He slumped down on the bed and buried his face in his hands.

"You would not understand. I had a very good hand. There was a pile of money on the table. I thought that if I won it, I would be able to buy you the moon... Oh, God, what am I to do now?" His hand-shrouded head sank down towards his knees. Molly could not bear to see him like this, defeated and depressed: he normally enjoyed such an irrepressible nature. The indomitable Englishwoman in her came to the fore.

"David, my love; go and get dressed. We are going to the Restaurant tonight, after all." Molly took charge.

"Molly, dearest: we cannot! I have told you we have lost... " David began but his wife cut across his protests.

"We shall discuss what we are going to do in the morning, but tonight, we shall show a brave face to the world in our adversity. None one must suspect we cannot afford to lose two thousand pounds. I have enough cash left from my monthly allowance to cover the cost of this meal, so we will go to the Restaurant and hold our heads high, for this evening at least. Now, will you please go and get ready: I think I have been kept waiting for long enough."

"Yes dear," assented David, and marvelled again at the strength of his wife's character. If he had known of her conversation of this afternoon, he might just have suspected she was trying to prove how she too could bear all manner of hardship in the support of her husband, like her friend, Lorna Wainwright.

News travels fast anywhere, but never as speedily as in the closed community of a ship. It seemed every head in the room craned around to take a lingering look at David and Molly as they walked into the à la carte Restaurant, hand in hand. No single person came forward to offer condolence or commiseration; rather, they shunned the fated couple like pariahs, in case close communication, or a casual touch, might impart some part of the bad luck which obviously dogged them.

The Maitre d' found them a table for two in the corner, out of the way, sensing the mood of his other patrons, and tried hard to put them out of his mind. Only their Steward, and the Wine Steward, approached them, offering deferential service, and they ate a pleasant, but solitary, meal in virtual isolation from the rest of the room. It was a far cry from the 'rubbing of shoulders with the titled' that David had originally intended. Yet Molly certainly played the part of the great lady to exaggeration, head held proudly high, giving her orders in a clear, haughty voice, even if David had not yet recovered from the drubbing he had received at the card table, or the uncharacteristic drinking bout he had indulged in afterwards. Molly kept a weather-eye on her husband, allowing him two glasses of wine with the food, but dispensing with the liqueurs when the coffee was served, which was their normal practice. She was completely in charge of the 'putting on a good face' ceremony, which was what this was all about: David being more like a sponge of attrition, still soaking up the damage he had done to the family finances, and his ego.

As they were preparing to leave, John Sayer turned up out of the blue - he must have been watching them, Molly concluded later.

"Hi there!" he greeted, flashing a warm smile at Molly, his eyes not failing to take in David's wilted condition. "Molly, ya better go and join my wife, an' the other ladies, in the Veranda Café. We'll see ya later, huh! Me an' your husband there, had better hev' a long, quiet talk." Molly could not possibly guess what this might be about, but Sayer's forceful manner did not brook trivial argument in any case, so she readily agreed. She did not see why she should cower away in her cabin. This affair was, after all, nobody's business but theirs.

"Where ve 'ell 'ave ya bin 'iding all day?" demanded Tom, when he met Sian that evening, as surreptitiously arranged.

"We couldn't exactly walk round 'oldin' hands wit' yer wife on board, could we?" retorted Sian.

"I've bin goin' bleedin' spare," grumbled Tom. "I didn't fink ya wanted ta see me agin. I nearly got ta pullin' me 'air aut."

"Whorr, after what yer did to me last night? I were only tryin' ter keep out the way: I didn't want ter get yer into trouble, like," she explained.

They were standing face to face; he looking down, and her up, plaintively. Her skin was smooth beside the turned-up nose, and a dusting of dark, brown freckles flecked her cheeks beneath the burnished, copper crown. Tom recalled how her flesh had felt last night, firm yet yielding, and how her soft, full lips had tasted. A fire started to rage in the pit of his loins.

"Ware's yer wife," Sian inquired, "luking after the kids, like?"

"Yas. Gorn ta bed most like!" Amy had shown no inclination to come out this evening, although she had begged Tom not to be late. It must be because she felt insecure: he did not believe she had any sexual aspirations. Amy was the least of his concerns at the moment.

"What are we gunna do abaut vis? I bin finkin' abaut ya every minute. I can't git ya outa me mind," he told her.

"I dunno! Whorr do yer want to do about it?" she rejoined. "Whorr if I'm up the spout, like? Yer didn't 'old back nuttin' last night." The women in Tom's experience were all very basic. He had never climbed above the bottom rung of the English class structure, so was not embarrassed by the question.

"We'll bouf 'ave ta give vat some serious fought," he suggested.

"While we're thinkin', like, 'ad we better 'ave a monkey dance," chuckled Sian. "The people round 'ere are beginnin' to take a good luke arrus."

"Yas," agreed Tom, and allowed himself to be led towards the tender mercies of the improvised band.

"I don't care what ya say! In all the years I've bin playin' poker, I cain't ever remember anyone drawin' three cards to fill up a runnin' flush," Sayer was saying. David sipped the large, neat brandy the Canadian had brought him; the smooth spirit comforting his crushed being. "What would a guy hold in a hand like that, two different cards of the same suit? If it had been a stripped deck, it might have bin worth a shot, but not in a full deck of fifty two cards. The chances of it coming up must be a billion to one!"

"And yet we all saw him turn over his cards," David reminded him. "It must have been his lucky day, that's all."

"What... against four aces? Have you any idea what the odds are of two hands like that coming out in a whole session, let alone in one game?" David realised Sayer was intimating something.

"What precisely are you suggesting?" he asked.

"I'm not suggestin' anythin', I'm tellin' ya! There's somethin' aboot Mr Lucas Meredith which is not quite right."

"Are you saying he cheated?" demanded David, and the Canadian stared at him meaningfully. "How would he do that?"

"Hundreds of ways!" Sayer told him. "Say... have ya got that deck of cards he gave ya, on ya?" David felt in his pockets. He could hardly remember taking them in the highly charged atmosphere at the end of the game, or transferring them to his dinner-jacket, but he must have, as he found them in his coat pocket.

"Yes... I have."

"Lemme see them, will ya," insisted Sayer, and David handed them over. He must be in a worse daze than he perceived.

Sayer examined the pack minutely; fanning out the cards in his huge hands, and running his finger-tips gently over the edges.

"What are you looking for?" David wanted to know.

"Lumps; bumps; marks; anythin'. I want to see if our friend Meredith was usin' a marked deck."

"But that's impossible! He opened a new pack at the commencement of the game. Don't you remember? He spread them out on the table for all to see." Sayer's pitying look made David feel like an idiot.

"And why would he want to do a thing like that, unless it was to make sure we trusted him: so no one would notice when he switched the pack," Sayer declaimed triumphantly.

"You think he switched the pack?" David exclaimed incredulously, but John Sayer did not reply immediately. He sorted out the contending hands, the aces and the run of diamonds; holding them up to the light, looking for tell-tale pinpricks.

"Yes," he said at length... although I don't see why... these cards are not marked in any way I can detect." He returned the pack to its original state and handed it to David. "Keep 'em," he advised, "just in case." Then he suddenly ejaculated, "The crafty bastard... he wanted you to have the cards so everyone could see they were not marked. He's a mechanic!"

David, still numb from the stinging pain in his burnt fingers, did not understand the Canadian's train of thought.

"What are you saying, John?"

"Don't ya see, bucko? He didn't use a marked deck at all. He set us all up. He paid the piper and we just danced to his toon." David was completely lost by Sayer's adage, but fortunately the Canadian was about to explain. "Look, he gits another pack from somewhere, the same, an' he arranges them to suit himself... so he has the whip-hand. When the time is right - when it's his deal - all he has to do is substitoot his loaded deck for the real one, and there it is. He deals us all a hand an' we play it, just how he wants, an' he's sittin' there knowin' what everybody in the game has." David was beginning to comprehend. "David, my boy, you have bin hit on by a card shark!"

"But when could he have changed packs? Surely, one of us would have seen him?" objected David, and then the light began to dawn on both of them.

"Remember, he had a coughing fit just before he dealt that hand."

"He said it was something to do with my cigar."

"Ideal time to switch packs; no one would have suspected."

"But what can I do?" complained David.

"Go see the Captain: he is the authority on this ship," suggested Sayer.

"I cannot go running to the Captain like a little boy! What shall I tell him? I've lost my money in a card game, sir, and could you get it back for me?" David uttered the words derisively. Sayer shrugged.

"If you can afford to lose that sort of money to a cheat, go ahead, but I know what I would do."

"Which is?"

"Stop the damn cheque, man, as soon as you get to New York! Better still, use the ship's facilities: cable your instructions ahead."

"I cannot do that: I gave my word," protested David.

"It's your money, but don't be a fool twice in one day." Sayer tried to dominate David then. "It ain't only your money. That guy took Poulson and Weidner too, for a deal of money on that hand. As the biggest loser, it's up to you to do somethin' aboot it, in case the guy decides to take some other sucker on this ship."

Suddenly, David was very angry to be regarded in those terms. He had been duped along with all the others: how could he have known? They certainly had not, at the time! Indignation at all the pain he had suffered at the hands of Lucas Meredith bubbled and boiled, like a volcano, inside him, until it vented itself through his throat.

"I ought to kill him," he mouthed angrily, and Sayer placed a restraining hand on his arm, feeling the young man's steely muscles flexing involuntarily.

"I don't think that's a good idea," he counselled. "Take my advice; go tell the Captain."

"No, I shall not run to the Captain," David stated adamantly. "There is an aphorism, where I come from, that 'God does not pay his debts in money', and Mr Meredith will get his just deserts before this voyage is over, I can tell you!"

"You know your own business best, but if you won't accept my guidance and see the Captain, I sure hope you won't do anythin' stoopid," advised Sayer soberly. "Now, I better buy ya another drink. I'm sure a lucky man to have escaped myself; that guy couldn'ta liked the colour of my money."

David was not prepared to say any more on the subject, although his mind teemed with sinister plans.

"What if... " he began. "What if one of us had not acted as predicted: taking more or less cards than Meredith anticipated, spoiling his little ploy?" he inquired.

"I guess he would have stacked his hand and waited for another opportoonity. Then the guy's a professional! Maybe, he had another surprise up his sleeve we'll never even know aboot." He studied David calculatedly. "Guys like Meredith ain't stoopid, son. He had plenty of time to probe us over the last coupla days... just you remember that!" The warning was implicit in the words.

When David rejoined Molly after the discussion, he had perked up, though cold ire had replaced the depression.

"I did not lose at cards," he proclaimed. "I was cheated; swindled out of my money."

"What are you going to do?" she inquired tentatively.

"Beard the lion in his den," he replied decisively, and nothing she could say would persuade him to change his mind. She noted that he was in a dangerous mood; she had never seem him this angry before.

The Second Officer heard the news by way of one of his juniors, who stopped for a gossip on the bridge on his way to bed. Instantly the face of the lonely card player, he had spotted in the First Class Smoking Room, slotted into place in his brain. He had seen the man before, on his previous ship, when one of the passengers was taken for a similar amount, in the same circumstances. There was nothing much he could do about it now, as he was on watch until ten, but he determined to do something as soon as he was able. He did not care for rogues and cheats! While he waited to be relieved, he searched his memory banks for the man's name, but it would not come. One thing was certain, however, it had not been Meredith, and to his mind, only people with something to hide changed their names.

He saw his chance when the Captain arrived on the bridge, straight from the dinner table, as was the Old Man's normal routine.

"Everything alright, Second?" he asked as he always did; meaning the functions of the ship.

"With the ship, yessir, but not, with the passengers, I'm afraid," reported the officer. The Captain sighed.

"What is it now?" He did not need aggravation on his last voyage, and there always seemed to be something ready to try his patience, when he was weary.

"I'm afraid we have a card shark on board, sir. One of the passengers has been swindled out of a great deal of money: in excess of two thousand pounds, I understand."

"Oh dear! Are you sure?" checked the Captain. These affairs could be very messy if not handled circumspectly, and he really did not want to know, not at present.

"Yes sir. I've seen the man before, on the *Majestic,* a couple of years ago. He did the same thing then, sir: took one of the passengers for a very large sum in fishy circumstances. There was a terrible shermozzle at the time. Apparently, the man had been working the Company's ships for some while: I understood him to be banned from the Line after the incident."

"I'm sure the Booking Office would not make that sort of mistake! As far as I am aware, they are most conscientious over black-listed passengers," demurred the Captain.

"I don't think they would have known, sir. The man is not travelling under his proper name... at least, it was not the name he was using on the *Majestic*. It speaks volumes, don't you think, sir?"

"It doesn't prove a thing," argued the Captain. "Are you completely sure it is the same man?"

"Yes sir. I recognised him instantly," declared the Second Officer recklessly; anxious to prove his point.

"Why the devil didn't you say something earlier?" growled the Captain. "We might have been able to stop this happening, if you had. Prevention is always better than a cure!" The Old Man did not sound very pleased and the Second Officer was left trying to regain his ground.

"Well sir, his face rang a bell... but I didn't twig who he was until I heard about the... "

"It's a pity you didn't 'twig' a lot earlier," reprimanded the Captain; he did not approve of modern idioms on his bridge. "You might have saved us all a great deal of trouble."

"Yes sir," replied the Second Officer; lamely shuffling his feet.

"What do you expect me to do about it, in any case?" demanded the Captain, and the Second Officer perked up again.

"I thought you might have the man up before you, sir... warn him off... make him give the money back. This sort of incident cannot be good for the Line!"

"I don't need you to tell me what is good for the Line," thundered the Captain. "I already have the Chairman on my back twenty-four hours a day: I don't require you to climb up there with him."

"No sir," muttered the officer contritely; dumbfounded. He had not intended, in his enthusiasm to see justice done, to say the wrong thing, or to sound in any way patronising. It was not turning out to be his day!

"Has there been any complaint?" asked the Captain in a more liberal tone, though the annoyance was still plain.

"No sir, not yet: not that I know of."

"Then I do not see there is a lot I can do; not tonight; not at this hour." The Captain thought for a minute, looking out through the bridge windows, his gaze fixed well ahead of the liner. He could think of a thousand such episodes in the past, both trivial and serious, and realised for the first time, how much he was going to miss everyday life aboard ship. Then he conjured up images of his grandchildren and perceived how he had also missed them growing up, and his own children, and felt it was time to put things right. "Second," he said. So many officers had served under him in his time, he preferred to use the title, not the name, to avoid confusion. It was a lot easier, especially now when his memory was not what it had been.

"Yes sir."

"Find out all you can about this business, and give me a full report in the morning. I will decide what is to be done then."

"Aye aye, sir."

"Goodnight Second." He suspended further discourse and forced back the apology, over the unreasonable outburst, which had sprung to his lips spontaneously. Good Captains do not apologise - junior officers must learn to take both censure and compliment in their stride if they wish to progress in the service - and he intended to be a good Captain until the moment he surrendered his command. He set off for his sleeping quarters: Sunday was always a busy day for him, and he would have to be up early. It looked like it might be even more full than usual.

"G'night, sir," the Second Officer called after him with respect in his voice.

A strong signal came into the Marconi Room at ten thirty pm. It was from the *Rappahannoch*, passing close by on her way east. She had sustained damage while coming though a field of pack ice, twenty-four hours before. She bleated out the plaintive morse warning for all and sundry to hear.

Harold Bride, the operator on duty, and despite his imagined difficulties, deduced it serious enough to warrant special attention. He abandoned his warm shack and carried the message-form to the bridge. The First Officer, who had taken over the watch, took the flimsy sheet into the chartroom and plotted the co-ordinates. The reported ice field was a long way off, almost a day's run, and twenty-four hours is a long time at sea: much can change in a day. He did not consider it serious enough to wake the sleeping Captain, or politic: the Old Man's temper was uncertain when roused from a sound sleep.

He left the message on the chart and returned to his duties on the bridge. The vagaries of the draughts from the constantly opening door, would consign the form to the floor, thence to the cleaner's basket and history!

The Second Officer tapped softly on the stateroom door, not really expecting the occupants to be up at this late hour. He was still incensed over the news of the swindle and felt it was his duty to push the Captain along the right path. If he could just get this man, who had obviously been duped, to complain, it would bring matters to a head nicely. His persistence was rewarded when the door swung open. A man in his mid-thirties, handsome under a mop of slicked-down ginger hair, filled the door frame, blocking any view of the interior of the cabin. He was dressed in a black dinner-jacket, appearing wide awake and hostile.

"What do you want?" David demanded.

"Mr Peacock?"

"Yes."

"I'm the Second Officer, sir. I came to tell you the man you played cards with today is a notorious card shark."

"I have just about managed to work that out for myself," snapped David, and the Second Officer was not surprised by his belligerence.

"Quite so. I came to advise you... well, if you would like to make a complaint to the Captain in the morning, I am sure something can be done to ensure you get your money back."

"Thank you, but no. I have made up my mind to deal with the 'gentleman' in my own way." The officer was alarmed: it sounded like a threat to him, and he could not countenance passengers taking the law into their own hands.

"I beg you to reconsider, sir," he began. "Making a complaint to the Captain is by far the best way to have the situation handled. Obviously, this is a common occurrence for us, and we do have the machinery to deal with it." Surprisingly, the man scoffed at him.

"Yes, and have my name bandied about the ship for a fool. No thank you! I am something of a laughing stock already, I have no doubt."

"No, sir," the officer denied sincerely. David continued.

"This affair is between the two of us, and will be settled in the manner of gentlemen. Now, I thank you for your concern and bid you goodnight." The Second Officer found the stateroom door securely slammed in his face.

He stood about in the gangway outside, uncertain what to do. He conjured up a mental image of the hot-headed Mr Peacock, and the gambler, facing each other across the poop-deck, in shirtsleeves, and with swords drawn in the dawn light. He decided to make sure the Master at Arms was fully conversant with what could turn into an ugly situation.

"There you are, dear," commented Molly as David turned back into the room.

"You see, you are not alone in this." She had heard every word which transpired, and feared for her husband's rationality in his present, affronted mood. She recognised it as a period when men were at their most dangerous.

"Hadn't you better take the officer's advice and see the Captain in the morning? I do not think it is a good idea to confront this Mr Meredith tonight." David stood stock still in the centre of the cabin; deep in thought.

"Come to bed and get some sleep," encouraged Molly. "We will take a fresh look at things in the morning." She lay on the bed enticingly, the peignoir slightly open to display her long, shapely legs. She felt so afraid for him, she would do anything to keep him here. It was no good: David was not about to be discouraged.

"Sleep! How can I sleep?" he charged, and began to pace up and down the cabin like a caged lion, as he had been doing before the interruption. "How can I ever sleep again, until I have resolved this?" he burst out dramatically. "How could I ever have been so cretinous as to allow myself to be set up, or fall for a trick like that!" It was his damaged ego which fired him up.

"It is not your fault... you could not have known... it could have happened to anyone." Molly uttered soothing platitudes in the hope of calming him down, but it was not to be. His agitated pacing was a means to screw up his courage for the showdown which must take place this very evening. If he did not do it now, he would never do it! Nor would his masculine obstinacy allow him to go running to the Captain with tales of being hard done by. He was a man, and must take care of his own affairs.

"It is my fault and I must put it right," he inveighed. "Wait there, my love: I must go." He turned his back and single-mindedly headed for the door.

"Don't go!" Molly called out to him, but he took no notice, slamming the door behind him in his purposefulness. "Please don't go, David. Please come back!" Molly continued to wail after him, fearful of what he might do, or what might happen to him.

Lucas Meredith had diplomatically taken dinner in his suite that evening. There was no point in aggravating his victim, who must be feeling pretty bloody by now. Besides, he needed to relax from the stress he suffered while perpetrating his coup. It was never easy to sit there executing one of the most despised acts known to the gambling fraternity; a time fraught with tension and imminent danger - one could never forecast what might happen if he had picked the wrong target. Now he lounged in an armchair, completely tranquil; wearing a plum-coloured, velvet smoking-jacket, with gaudy, satin-paisley lapels: a weakness of his. A long, thin cheroot burned between his graceful fingers, and the latest novel by H Rider Haggard lay open on his lap. He remembered his favourite author had been knighted in the Honours List that very year, and wished the title he assumed, from time to time, might have been genuine. If his gambling career in the casinos of Europe had not been so sadly terminated, he might well have become rich enough to buy one by donating the correct amount to the right party's funds. It would not be the case now, and he would have to be content with his play acting, although it would never be the same. The coins and notes he had won this afternoon, had long since been stashed in the false bottom of his solitary suitcase - he travelled light - along with the cheque, and it was concern for this which obliterated his concentration in the elegant prose in front of him. He did not like cheques, preferring to have the security of cash.

There came a tap at the door but it did not alarm him unduly. He was expecting the Steward, with the bedtime cup of cocoa he had ordered, and called out, "Come in." A second later, a deranged-looking David Peacock had burst into the room and was standing over him. Lucas leapt to his feet in terror, narrowly avoiding head-butting the man; the book falling to the deck, at his feet, with a thud which made him jump. It looked like Lucas was about to attack, and David backed off; an action which would not help his cause. Lucas was, suddenly, very afraid, and his heart thumped rapidly against his ribcage. The hideous mask of rage which faced him was very different from the placid features he had encountered earlier in the day. The man had been drinking; Lucas could smell the bouquet on his breath - and he wondered if his selection system had failed him at last, and if he was about to face his Armageddon. He did not drink himself but had seen many times before just what it could do to a man, especially an aggrieved one.

"What the devil?" he ejaculated. "What do you mean by bursting in here...? Get out this instant."

"No," replied David coldly. "You invited me to come in. As to why I burst in here: I want my cheque back. You can keep the cash you won off me - I will put that down to experience - but I want my cheque."

"Get out," Lucas repeated.

"You are a cheat, sir; a rogue and a charlatan," David continued high-handedly. "You took my money by the foulest means available and I intend to have it back."

"I don't know what you are talking about," submitted Lucas as a defence. David stepped forward and snatched the cheroot out of the gambler's fingers. "You see, even your no-smoking ruse is an absolute fraud." David dropped the cheroot onto the carpet and ground it out viciously with his heel. Lucas faced his tormentor bravely. Much of his life had contained strife: it came with the territory. "I even know how it was done," David railed on. "I worked it out for myself. You obtained a spare pack, arranged the cards as you wished, then dealt it to us; saving the best hand for yourself."

"You prove it," Lucas rejoined, cockily. He had already disposed of the incriminating cards.

"I do not have to prove anything! We both know you cheated me!" snarled David.

"And a fat lot of good that will do you. There are no policemen on board, you know," returned Lucas.

"I do not need a policeman," David informed him. "I intend to stay here, in your cabin, until you return my cheque and the money you extorted from Mr Poulson and Mr Weidner. I think you will become fed up with my unpleasant company long before I do!"

Lucas relaxed and was no longer afraid. He was not about to be attacked or it would have happened by now: the man was a windbag! He recalled how David had backed away when he stood up. David Peacock had position, and his wife and children on board with him. He could not afford to do anything rash which might jeopardise his standing, or embroil himself in a nasty situation. Lucas could rely on the English to keep calm, control their tempers, and do the right thing: it was the hot-blooded foreigners one had to watch! He went over to the attack.

"You are wasting your time... now get out," he uttered intrepidly. David shook his head.

"No. You invited me in. I do not intend to leave until you have returned my cheque, as I said before."

"I could call the Master at Arms," suggested Lucas.

"Call him," challenged David. "Call who you like. I have nothing to hide if you wish to air this affair in public... whereas I know you have. One of the officers has recognised you, and knows you for what you are." Lucas did not bat an eyelid. For two pins, David would have smashed the gambler's features to pulp - he was big, strong, and fit enough to do it - but he remembered John Sayer's words of caution, and reluctantly restrained himself.

Lucas turned and strode away across the stateroom; decorated and furnished in Queen Anne style. When he turned back and faced David from a few feet away, a supercilious grin was stamped on his ruggedly handsome features.

"David Peacock, prominent businessman, from London most likely: a member of several clubs. Am I right?" he inquired. When David said nothing, Lucas continued. "It would not be very hard to verify when I return to London; I have some good contacts in the city. So do your damnedest, my friend. Threaten me, stay here as long as you like, stop the cheque you have given me, which is what you are going to do if I don't return it, isn't it?" Still David did not reply. He stared at Lucas, as if hypnotised by a dangerous serpent, ill prepared for what was to come. Lucas went on mercilessly. "How would it be if your associates, and fellow club members, were to learn you welshed on your bets? What price the lofty Mr Peacock then? I would show the cheque around, of course. A dishonoured cheque would be a powerful banner to parade about the town, and I will, I make no bones about it! No one would ever doubt a man of your experience and acumen had owed me the money, or the cheque would never have been written in the first place, and your signature is quite clear: I examined it very closely before I put the cheque away in a place you will never find in a month of Sundays, and nor will anyone else, for that matter. You can say whatever you like about me, of course - sticks and stones and all that - but I must warn you: mud sticks, whatever the truth of the matter concerned. I know, believe me: it has been a cross I have had to bear all my life."

"You... you bloody swine!" David stormed in despair. He knew Meredith was telling the truth: he had witnessed several men ruined in this way, ostracised and never trusted again, for reneging on their gambling debts.

"No, I am not," protested Lucas. "I am a business man, like yourself, and always prepared to offer an arrangement beneficial to all parties concerned." He looked David up and down. "What I propose is quite fair to both of us. I do not like cheques, and I am not a greedy man. When we arrive in New York, you will go to your bank and draw out half the disputed amount, in cash; say twelve hundred pounds. When you deliver this cash to my hotel, I will return your cheque, and we can both go our separate ways. No tricks, mind: I have seen them all before. How does that sound? Do we have an agreement?" He still thought David was a wealthy man, and was prepared to cut his losses for the sake of securing cash, and he had won enough to suit his present needs from the other two patsies. He did not know twelve hundred pounds was more, much more, than David could afford.

"I ought to bloody-well horsewhip you for your cheek!" snapped David, and Lucas grinned.

"Oh, I would not even consider such an action, Mr Peacock, if I were you. The pain would blur my memory, and I might well forget just where it was I hid your cheque... Well, do we have an agreement?"

"I will have to give the matter some serious thought," stated David, trying to stave off the inevitable; seeing himself trapped in a cleft stick.

"Take all the time you need: we still have four days of the voyage to go," said Lucas magnanimously. "But I warn you, my offer is only valid for twenty-four hours after we dock in New York. After that, I shall pay your cheque into my bank for presentation at yours. It will either have to be met, or I shall look forward to seeing the little remark, in red ink, 'refer to drawer', on that expensive paper. I take it you catch my drift?" Lucas was quite enjoying himself. "Now, get out of my stateroom... I wish to go to bed."

The party in the steerage area broke up early. It became bitterly cold as the hour grew late, and the revellers drifted away piecemeal, looking for warm beds. The band struggled on for a while to accommodate the hardy few who remained, but the cold stiffened fingers and snatched at the breath, until they too were forced to give up. If they had been paid for their efforts, like the orchestra in the Palm Court, it might have been a different story, but there is no point in playing for pleasure when there is none.

Tom and Sian, having no bed to go to, and being deprived of the warmth provided by the rapid movements of the strenuous dances, retired to a dark corner to wait for the ship to retire. They cuddled close, but even so, felt the chill beginning to gnaw at their bones.

"Blimey, gel, I'm wore aut already, and we ain't done nuffin yet," Tom was complaining.

"Don't you think of anythin' else?" Sian reproved.

"What else is ver ta fink about?" he replied and winked at her knowingly.

"We don't know anytin' about each other, like. What do yer do for a livin'?"

It seemed an odd question to Tom just at this moment.

"I'm a chippy." She looked at him uncertainly. "I'm a carpenter, like," he clarified, and her face lit up.

"Me uncle says there's a lorra building wurk goin' on in Chicago. You shouldn't 'ave any trouble gerrin a job up thurr." Here was the enticement again, and the fabled uncle of hers seemed to know everything about everything.

"I already gotta job, see, with me bruver; in New York," Tom told her.

"Please yerself," returned Sian, not a little put out. "Yer can wurk where yer like!"

"Come on, gel, don't be like vat," Tom demurred.

"Well, you men are all the same. You lead a girl on to get 'er body, and then once you've 'ad it, yer don't want to know no more. I thought yer cared fur me, like."

"I do, gel, I do," Tom assured her. "I fink I'm in love whiff ya."

"Whorr are yer goin' to do about it, then? You know I might be up the stick after last night."

"I dunno. I've got me wife an' kids ta consider."

"Yer didn't consider them, last night, when yer were pokin' it up me, like," protested Sian. "You came along and swept me off me feet, and made me fall in love wit yer, and now you've had yer fun, yer wanna go runnin' back to yer wife."

"Naw, it ain't like vat at all: ya know it ain't," Tom rubbished her sentiments. "It's just... well... what am I gonna do abaut vem, vat's all. I mean, I can't just tell vem to bugger orf, can I: I've sold their 'ome and brought vem to America whiff me. What are vey goin' ta do if I ain't vere."

"That's your problem, if yer wanna be wit' me, like," Sian told him.

"I do wanna be whiff ya, ya know vat, it's just what's gonna 'appen to vem, see."

"You go back to wifey, then," Sian told him petulantly. "I've gorra go to me bed."

Sian pulled away from him, and made as if to leave, but he grabbed her around the body, with his long arms, and held her in a bearhug, close to him.

"Naw, gel, ya ain't goin' like vat. Ya gotta give me a coupla days to fink abaut it. I do love ya; ya know I do. Naa, let's find a nice, warm place: it's gettin' bleedin' chilly up 'ere." Sian had not yet finished with him.

"Just like a man," she grumbled. "Yer want yer cake and eat it. Yer want to poke that dirty thing of yours up me while yer decide if yer goin' ter leave the missus, like. Well, I'm norr 'aving that!" She began to struggle and squirm in his arms and he had to use all his strength to hold her.

"Alright, alright, calm darn, for Chrissake! I'm whiff ya, gel, ain't I? Ya gotta give me a coupla days ta get used to ve idea, ain't ya? I mean, we don't want no trouble on board, do we? An' if Amy finds aut, she'll flay ve bleedin' 'ide orf ya." Sian gave up her struggle. "Naa, let's go an' find some place warmer ta talk, gel: if we stays up 'ere any longer, me nuts will drop orf and ven where will we be, hey?" It was Sian's turn to be led towards the companionway.

Deep down below, they found the same indolent steward had left the Linen Room open again, and they crept in there quietly as they had the night before. There would be no further talk. The kissing started, but in a much more deliberate way, and the subtle movements against each other, and the wandering palms, were better controlled. Tom's hands found their way into her blouse and through the camisole, somehow; cupping her tip-tilted, half-melon breasts and feeling for the hard, sharp nipples. Sian tugged at his belt, fighting to free it from the buckle, and Tom drew in his stomach muscles to help her. Their passion became urgent, and Tom released a hand to pull up her long skirt; running his fingers over the soft flesh of her inner thighs, seeking to clear away the prohibitive underclothes. She was not wearing any, and he drew in his breath sharply as his hand contacted her warm, wet quim. Sian had freed him from his breeches, and he lifted her up onto one of the lower shelves, at the right height, cushioned by the crisp linen, so he could enter her. Sian tucked her long legs out of harm's way and guided him to the portals of her inner self, with a soft, satiny hand; watching him closely as he pushed himself in, half closing his eyes in ecstasy.

She continued to watch closely as he drove into her faster and faster, as if waiting for the right moment. He managed to prolong his ardour tonight, cleaving her apart in a steady cadence, which sucked and slopped in the vacuum of her juices. Sian waited - unconcerned with enjoyment - until he began to moan, his stabbing becoming frantic, while he rode up on her loins, as high as he could reach.

"Oh... oh... oh," she cried in mock culmination. "Yer will come to Chicago wit' me, won't yer, Tom? Tell me yer will... tell me yer will."

"Yas... yas... yas... " Tom roared in rhythm with his appendage, as he thrust it in uncontrollably, and Sian relaxed, with a superior-looking smile on her face, allowing him to spray his essence all over her core.

SUNDAY 14th APRIL 1912

The Captain rose early and was on the bridge at dawn. There was nothing in the clear skies, the flat sea, or the slight haze which hung over the water, beyond the huge windows of the bridge, that led him to believe it was a significant one. Apart from the unfortunate collision while commanding the *Olympic*, his career had been remarkably untroubled, and untoward thoughts of disaster never entered his head. The only sensation he felt was the cold, and he snuggled into his greatcoat thankfully, turning his attention to the day's work.

His concerns over the coal bunker fire had diminished - there had been no further reports to cause concern - although his stricture with regard to its sealing had not been rescinded. Perhaps, he thought to himself, he had been somewhat old-womanish over his approach to the affair but then Captain's need not explain themselves, and shortly, he would no longer have to worry about such things. Most commanders had their idiosyncrasies and he was no exception: a fire on board had always been one of his obsessions. He knew then, the thing which would please him most in retirement - apart from his grandchildren - was the concept of spending what life he had left without being constantly watched, appraised, and looked up to, as he had been for as long as he could remember. The notion he would no longer be expected to set an example, or to watch his every word and deed, or behave diplomatically, pleased him immensely; he could appear at dinner dressed solely in his tropical shorts, if he so desired, and his patient wife would be the only one able to criticise him. If there was much he would gain by the move, there was also a great deal he would lose: absolute power, a crew's respect, the feeling of importance - all of which had been a drug to him in his younger days, but he had come to terms with it by now and made peace with his motivation.

In the absence of an amenable clergyman on board, he would conduct Divine Service in the First Class Dining-Room after breakfast. Any passenger who so desired would be permitted to attend - God, unlike man, made no distinction - and all the physical barriers, the latticed steel gates, between the First, Second and Third

Class portions of the ship, would be unlocked for the duration of the rite. The Captain enjoyed these none too frequent moments of simple worship; feeling it brought him closer to Our Lord than the sanctimonious hypocrisy of many of the frocked ministers he had encountered, who could not distinguish sincerity from cant. It was the last time he would be privileged to serve God in this way, and was another detail he regretted about his impending retirement.

At nine am, a message was received in the wireless room from the Cunard Liner *Caronia*, reporting an ice field, containing growlers and icebergs, in latitude 42 North, from longitude 49 to 51 West. The warning was passed to the bridge, and the plot put the hazard some three hundred and fifty miles ahead. It was not considered to be of great importance at the time. Visibility was good and icebergs were common at this time of year, as the pack ice in Northern Canada around Hudson Bay broke up and drifted south. Many ships threaded their way through this detritus every day, and it was not regarded as dangerous, as long as a good look-out was kept. The *Titanic* had two men constantly on watch in the crows-nest. Among the officers and crew, all was tranquil.

Two of the passengers were not so calm; Tom Pirbright and David Peacock. Tom had woken beside Amy, the air heavy and stale with exhaled carbon dioxide which the overworked air conditioning system had not been able to clear. He felt languid and listless, his limbs not wanting to move, and he was not sure if it was the effect of oxygen starvation or the exertions of last night which denied him energy. All he knew was, he would rather have woken up next to Sian. Amy stirred when he did, trying to turn towards him and elbowing him painfully in the chest as she did so.

"Whassa time?" she mumbled.

"Early... go back ta sleep." Tom told her exasperatedly. He was wide awake. He put his arms behind his neck, to prop up his head, and examined his wife. She surely looked mountainous beside the slender Sian. Now the thrill of passion had left him, he still did not know if he could do as he had promised; abandon Amy and run off to Chicago. He had told the girl he would, but the loyalty engendered by five years of marriage, and the birth of three children, was a powerful draw. He would wrestle with his conscience for most of the day. It was true Sian gave him delights Amy no longer could, or would, but he recognised his wife had three kids to contend with and could not be a sex goddess in the time she had left over from their care: it was a full time job. It was he who had brought her to this pass, taking his pleasure without regard for the consequences, and now he had betrayed her with a flibbertigibbet who had waved her arse at him. How long would it be, he wondered, before Sian had a clutch of kids by him, and ended up the same, overweight and constantly fatigued for her pains? Then there was the consideration that she had stolen one woman's man already, and what was to stop her doing it again when she tired of him? She was asking him to give up all for her: wife, children, family, security; while she was losing nothing to gain all. It hardly seemed a fair bargain to him. He wished, for a moment, he had never laid eyes on her, then remembered her throbbing body beneath him, last night, and was glad that he had. It was a big step to take, and required a lot of trust on his part. The painful soul searching, and the uncertainty, began all over again.

David Peacock sought to sweat out his anger and frustration in the gym. He worked very hard at the apparatus, especially the rowing machine, looking for relief, but the strenuous exercise had the opposite effect. It pumped up his muscles to their full strength and toned his powerful frame to good effect, until he felt like he could rip off his tormentor's arms and legs, then push his bleeding torso through a porthole into the sea below, closely followed by his limbs. He was embittered enough to do it. He could see why his forebears resorted to duels: a quick exchange of shots on a fresh morning would either resolve the problem or see to it that one was not in a position to brood over it further. That was the worst part about this: the languishing, being in limbo while one decided how to take revenge. Meredith may have thought he had gone off with his tail between his legs last night, but it was far from the truth. David had no intention of doing any deals over money he had been cheated out of and he could see no point in further argument. If Meredith was not prepared to return his cheque, he had plenty of time to find a way to retrieve it; now he could not risk having it stopped by the bank.

Molly's reaction, when he returned to the stateroom, had surprised him.

"Oh well, it's better than nothing," she had told him. "At least we will not be penniless as you feared. We will just have to do without our holiday and return home when your business is done. We will have to live circumspectly for the year, but I do not suppose it will do us any harm; we do live rather well, you know. It will be our little penance!" Twelve hundred pounds was not an excessive sum to shell out ensuring David was safely back in her arms uninjured, and without any serious charges hanging over his head - to her mind - but it was not a price David would pay for the same view. He determined not to tell Molly about his future plans, or seek further advice from the likes of John Sayer; presenting the final conclusion to this affair as a fait accompli. He did not set out to deceive her, only to be a bit frugal with the truth if she questioned him.

Lorna Wainwright had only just finished dressing her girls, in their Sunday best, for the morning service. Looking as pretty as a pair of Gainsborough portraits, their blonde hair flowing down over bright-blue, matching dresses, the girls sat quietly and watched their mother's preparations, in awe of the mysteries of grown-up women. Jonathan, by his calling, was an atheist, and had no truck with celestial myths; believing God was another word for the achievements of man. He had left to take a turn around the deck and would meet his family later, when their praying was done. Lorna was not going on her own: she had arranged to go with her new found friend, and would be collected herself, when Molly came to collect her children.

It was Molly who appeared to have the problems, when Lorna opened the door to her knock. Her eyes were red-rimmed, as if she had been crying, and her complexion was pale, bloodless, drained.

"Why, whatever is the matter, Molly dear?" Lorna asked as soon as she took in her friend's condition. "Are you feeling unwell?"

"No," denied Molly, "it is just that I have not slept very well."

"Are you sure?" persisted Lorna, fully concerned, and feeling guilty over being bright-eyed and bushy-tailed herself; a state she felt she owed to this woman's intervention in her life, and her kindness. "It looks considerably worse than that to me. Please tell me: I'm sure I could help. That is what friends are for." Molly gazed about her uncertainly, wide-eyed and disturbed, but the children were the only witnesses, and by tradition not there unless required, so she decided, at last, to unburden her heart. Once started, her troubles and distress bubbled out of her unabated. Lorna listened in consternation. Her Jonathan would never have taken such a risk: percentages to him were of much more importance. Perhaps Molly's suggested swap, even on a temporary basis, was not such a good idea after all!

"Perhaps this was what my forebodings were about," Lorna offered as a panacea to her friend, "and should we not go and thank God it was not a lot worse, like the ship sinking or something?" Her words were meant well, but did not give Molly much comfort.

The Chairman confronted the Captain on his way to hold morning worship.

"What's this I hear, about someone being cheated while playing cards?" demanded the Chairman. "Do you know anything about it?"

"Yes, I've had a full report from the Second Officer, this morning." The Captain did not perceive it was the Chairman's place to interfere in what was an internal matter, as far as he was concerned.

"Well, what do you intend to do about it?"

"There is not a lot I can do: I have received no complaint from the person concerned," the Captain informed him.

"Do you need a complaint? Can you not take action off your own bat? You are the supreme authority aboard this ship!" The Captain smiled wryly. He had believed the Chairman to be that.

"What do you think I should do: make the person responsible walk the plank? The day of clapping people in irons is long since gone, I'm afraid."

"You could start off by not being flippant," growled the irascible Chairman.

"This is not a good advertisement for the Line."

The Captain checked his watch. He detested being late for anything, especially not when there were many people waiting on him. With the other affairs of the ship pressing on his time, he had cut leaving the bridge very fine as it was.

"What do you expect me to do?" he repeated wearily.

"Well, at least give the chap one of your famous dressing-downs. We cannot have this sort of thing upsetting the passengers. Bad for business... bad for business." The Chairman shook his head dolefully, as if expecting the worst to come out of this.

"Very well," capitulated the Captain, without further argument, which he considered a waste of time when the overbearing Chairman was involved. "I will attend to it later, when I have time."

"I'd suggest sooner rather than later to be the best course. We cannot have this chap thinking he might get away with what he has done, and start all over again on some other unsuspecting soul."

"No, indeed," began the Captain, and finished the sentence more than sarcastically, "but then I can hardly summon this man and give him a tongue lashing in front of the Christian worshippers at Divine Service, whither I was bound when you stopped me. I do not think that would be good advertising for the Line in any shape or form!" His tone changed to one of forbidding solemnity; the type of verbalisation he used when addressing errant junior Officers. "I will deal with the matter in my own way as soon as I am able... as and when my more important duties allow... Good morning, sir," and he walked away, leaving the Chairman standing speechless behind him.

Thomas Andrews continued to haunt the ship, gliding from stem to stern, with notebook clutched in hand, checking here and there continuously. From the ornate timepiece in the First Class Lounge to the giant reciprocating engine, every mechanical system on the liner was working like clockwork. And yet, Andrews still filled his book with copious notes. To the uninitiated, they might have seemed petty points he faithfully recorded - this panel did not have sufficient screws; this support needed to be strengthened - but to him they had every importance. It was a chance to see the design he had inherited at work, and the time to spot necessary modifications, in field conditions, which would serve to improve the *Britannia*, still under construction at Harland and Wolff, if it was at all possible. As the *Titanic* had benefitted from the *Olympic's* early voyages, so would the *Britannia* advance to greater proficiency when it was her turn to set sail. Andrews laboriously transferred every detailed notation he made to a large blueprint of the ship he kept in his cabin, and spent hours poring over it, when he was not doing his rounds, on the table which had been specially installed. The *Titanic's* welfare was never far from his mind. It was a good job really; Lord Pirrie, the Chairman of Harlands, had been taken ill before the voyage: his role aboard would have only been a social one, and this wealth of information would never have emerged. Thomas Andrews was well satisfied with his labours.

At eleven-forty that morning, another message came into the Marconi Room. It was from the Dutch liner *Noordam*, reporting much ice at the same Latitude as the *Caronia*. Both operators were on standby, expecting Cape Race to be in range some time in the near future. When it was, their work could begin, and would not end until the mountain of messages, as presently held, had been cleared. Even then, there would be no real respite. Fingers, tired from tapping out morse code, would have to fumble back through the transmitted forms: weary brains, trying to shake off the tinnitus induced by buzzing headphones, would have to work out the cost of each message, so these could be passed to the Purser for charging to the senders' accounts. The wireless room staff would earn a fortune for their employers on this voyage but it was just a lot of hard work to Phillips and Bride. Phillips sent Bride, with the warning, to the bridge.

The officers were assembled for the daily sight as usual. The Captain was not present, so the Chief Officer took charge. The daily run was calculated - five hundred and forty-six miles since noon on Saturday; the best day's run yet. The position of the reported ice-field was also plotted, and was estimated to be two hundred and ninety miles ahead; fourteen hours running time for the ship. It might well drift a number of miles in that period so was not treated with any concern by the assembled officers.

The Captain was pacing up and down the deck of his day cabin. He had sent the Master at Arms to collect the gambler and was awaiting his return. These affairs unnerved him, as they always had. They distracted him from his real duties which was never a good thing aboard ship. If it had not been for the Chairman's intervention, he might well have let the incident pass by, despite the Second Officer's determination to have the culprit bought to book. Yet, as Captain, he must be seen to be doing the right thing, and would continue to practise this philosophy right up until the moment of his retirement. There came a knock at the door, and the Captain resigned himself to his unwanted task.

The man shown in by the Master at Arms was not what he had expected at all. Tall and elegantly dressed, with an almost military bearing, Lucas Meredith looked every inch the gentleman he had studied hard to portray. He did not look the least concerned at being brought here, summarily; as if he knew he had nothing to hide. Lucas had been through this scenario many times before, and knew the ropes expertly. He did not even think about what he would say - it was ingrained in his photographic memory - and never failed to issue from his mouth spontaneously. He looked at the Captain expectantly, aware he was causing the man to be uncomfortable. The Captain cleared his throat and began.

"It has... er... come to my attention that one of the passengers has lost a great deal of money in a card game in which you were also involved." Lucas framed the word 'so' with his mouth but it was never uttered. "Of course, the Line does not like this sort of thing: it does nothing for our reputation, you understand." Lucas made himself look bewildered.

"No, I don't understand: just what are you trying to convey to me?" The Captain started again.

"The card game in which you played, and won heavily, yesterday, has been called into question. It would seem that things were not quite right."

"What are you suggesting... that I cheated?"

"In a word, yes," the Captain said unhappily. Lucas allowed himself a controlled explosion.

"How dare you! I have never before been called a cheat... in my life. People who cannot afford to gamble should not do so! Nor should they come running to the authorities when they lose. Who has said this about me...? I've a good mind to sue."

"No one, yet: there has been no complaint," the Captain informed him.

"Then how can you listen to these foul accusations against me if there has been no complaint? Just because some people have sour grapes over losing in a fair game, what gives you the right to have me brought up before you, to suffer false allegations? I must protest most bitterly, and will complain, personally, to the Chairman of this Line when I return to England! I have never been insulted like this before, on any shipping line, and I shall see to it something is done to redeem my honour, if I have to go to law to do it!"

Lucas played the outraged gentleman exceptionally well, but it did not unduly impress the Captain. He had seen the like before.

"I don't think that to be the case. I think you have been insulted before, many times, in the same situation as this." Lucas looked at the Captain askance: his outraged indignation had cut no ice there. "For your information," continued the Captain, "the Chairman of the Line is on board: it is he who told me to have you up before me."

"Well, in that case..." Lucas began but was cut short.

"Mr Meredith, we are both well-travelled men of the world. Let's stop buggering about!" He reverted to bluff sailor's language. "Let me just say, before you go any further with your convincing charade, that you have been recognised by my Second Officer. He was serving on the *Majestic* when you did a similar thing: won a great deal in a suspect card game. He understood you had been banned from the Line over the incident." Lucas had overlooked the officers in his homework, so was not surprised, yet the expression on his face was one of incredulity.

"I have never been on that ship in my life... I have never been banned from any Line. This is an outrage, sir, to accuse me of this, especially when you have no proof, and no complaint has been received..." Lucas appeared to fall in.

"Oh... I see... this is a case of mistaken identity. How long is it since your officer served on this *Majestic?* I can prove I have never been on that ship. This is the first time I have ever left England. You will find he has mistaken me for another man whom I must resemble. How would the Booking Office have accepted my booking if I was banned from the Line? It is scandalous to treat innocent passengers in this fashion." The Captain had to admit his protestations were very good, his explanations first class, and wavered for a moment, almost convinced the man was right, and the Second Officer might be wrong. Then, he realised the man was just too good in his answers, too contrived to be genuine. The Second was right: this man was undoubtedly a cardsharp, working the ship.

"The Booking Office accepted you because you changed your name," he told Lucas deliberately; tired of this play acting.

"Changed my name... changed my name!" cried out Lucas almost hysterically. "My name is one of the proudest possessions of my family: my ancestors would all turn over in their graves if I did so. I tell you, your officer is mistaken... I mean, you look like my uncle, Lord Fawley, but I would hardly castigate him for losing this ship, if such a disaster occurred, just because of the resemblance." The Captain sighed deeply.

"Enough," he snapped. "I must own up: you are very good, but the fact remains you are a cheat and a liar, and I will not have your like aboard my ship. If you are as innocent as you say, and have never left England's shores before, how is it you know the Booking Office does not accept banned passengers? Why did you say 'you had been brought up before me' if you had not heard that particular expression before: it is naval jargon, not widely used outside the service. No, Mr Meredith, I do not believe you to be as innocent as you say, but must confess it is your lucky day."

"But I... " began Lucas.

"Shut up and listen!" thundered the Captain. "For I have had enough of your protestations and do not intend to repeat myself over and over again just to make my point." He continued in a normal voice. "It is your lucky day for no complaint has been received by me, about you, or I would have had you locked up in a storage cupboard for the remainder of the voyage. As it is, you will be watched, and there will be no recurrence of this deception: there will be no more card games, you understand. If I was you, I would confine yourself to your cabin until we reach New York. If I see your face again, I might be tempted to reverse my decision about that storage cupboard... Do I make myself clear?"

"I have never heard anything so offensive in my life. I shall consult my solicitor the moment I return to London and you, and your Chairman, will find yourself facing a very determined slander suit. Do I make myself... clear?" mocked Lucas, defiant to the bitter end.

"Consult who you like!" snapped the Captain, knowing it would never happen, and added, "Now get out!" He went to the door to call the Master at Arms.

The next ice warning came into the wireless room just after one pm. The message was written down and delivered to the Captain personally, back on the bridge after his encounter with Lucas Meredith. He read it briefly, and then handed it to one of his junior officers.

"Plot that for me, will you, Fourth? I want to know how far it is from our present position."

"Yes sir," gurgled the young man, pleased to be given the responsibility, and he hurried away to the chart-room. The Captain stared ahead, out of the bridge windows, as he waited for the report.

He was on his way to lunch, about one thirty, when he ran into the Chairman for the second time that day. The Chairman greeted him warily, recalling the disdain with which he had been treated earlier: the Old Man appeared to be a bit liverish today. The two men stopped for a brief chat. Surprisingly, the Captain's mood had changed, and he seemed quite affable now; full of pride over the performance of his ship.

"We made five hundred and forty six miles today; the best day's run on the voyage so far," he announced. "Very encouraging, don't you think?"

"Yes... very," concurred the Chairman. "The weather has been exceptionally clement. It is hardly surprising we are making good time."

"If it remains unchanged, I think we should bring her up to full speed for a short time tomorrow. It should be a good test. I am hoping she would make as much as twenty three knots, which should bode well for your ambition to wrest the Blue Riband away from the present holder, although I shall not be around to see it."

"Yes, it sounds like a good idea. However, you will inform Thomas Andrews, won't you? I am sure he would be more than pleased to see the ship at 'full throttle', so to speak, and his observations might be helpful for the future." So they circled around each other with swords at the ready, waiting for the other to move first: the Captain refusing to bring up the gambler, and knowing the Chairman was dying to ask but was obstinately waiting for him to report.

"Of course! I wouldn't dream of doing anything else," the Captain replied.

"What about the fi... our other little problem?" the Chairman wanted to know.

"I am pleased to report we have had no further indication that it is still alight. I think we can safely assume it is out."

"Good... Good." The Chairman held back any remarks which he felt might censure the Captain for his over-caution. He wished relations to return to normal. "Have you anything else to tell me?"

"No I don't think so," the Captain prevaricated. "Oh yes... I've had this message. I think you might be interested." The Chairman took the flimsy he was handed and glanced at the text. It was from the steamer *Baltic*. It read: 'Greek steamer *Athinai* reports passing icebergs and large quantities of field ice today in Latitude 41 51'N, Longitude 49 52' W. Wish you and the *Titanic* all success.' It was written in Jack Phillips' sloping capitals.

"Is this serious?" the Chairman asked.

"Good heavens, no... only routine. The ice field is two hundred and fifty miles ahead. It will probably not even be there when we arrive at that latitude. The Labrador Current is a powerful one. It will have swept the ice down the eastern seaboard of the continent by then."

"I hope you are right."

"I assure you, there is no need to be alarmed. We keep a very good look-out at all times, especially after such warnings." The Captain looked at his watch. "If you will excuse me, I will cut along to lunch. I have things to do this afternoon and I do not like to be late."

"Quite... quite," agreed the Chairman.

The Captain turned and took a few steps before he stopped and turned back.

"By the by, I have had a word with our friend, the gambling man... the card sharp. I don't think we will be hearing any more out of him."

"Good... good," commented the Chairman, but to himself. The Captain had turned away again and was hurrying down the Promenade Deck. The Chairman was left staring after him once more; the message from the *Baltic* still clutched in his hand. He folded it up and casually slipped it into his coat pocket.

Sunday was always a quiet day aboard ship, as the passengers followed pursuits adapted by the occasion. The chefs excelled themselves in the preparation of lunch; roasting great slabs of beef and pork, and succulent cuts of lamb, to be served with the traditional trimmings. Most of the older passengers retired to their cabins for a nap after lunch, as they might do at home, and only the young indulged in the pleasures afforded by the ship, keeping their activities circumspect out of respect for the Lord. There was no fixed routine or established recreational endeavours; even the staff of instructors and safety guards must have their time off, and Sunday was the best day to give it to them. Anyone who was rowdy, or overactive, would be considered ill bred, and looked down upon from then on, which was considered to be punishment enough. The remaining hours of daylight would pass uneventfully.

Another ice warning was intercepted from the liner *Amerika* at one forty-five, but Phillips was having a meal and Bride was alone in the Marconi Room. Such was the frequency of these messages, and the apparent lack of concern on the bridge, that young Harold did not see it as a priority and sidelined it for later delivery, when Phillips returned. In the flood of fresh messages which was about to come from the Purser's Office, it would be forgotten and never delivered to the officer on watch.

The Chairman held one of his soirées for the wives of some of the prominent passengers in the First Class Lounge at teatime. Most of them were American, including a Mrs Arthur Ryerson and Mrs Sayer, the wife of John. Hoping to impress their husbands, through them, with his hospitality, he had ordered many delicacies besides the traditional English fare: chocolate and walnut muffins, iced fancies, and the finest selection of delectable cakes the bakery had been able to provide. Some of the ladies picked at the goodies, while others wolfed them down, as the Chairman struggled to fabricate suitable small talk. It was always difficult for him; he was not a ladies man.

He latched onto one of his friends, the English Lady, and tried to hide behind her, taking the lead from what she said to keep the conversation going. The redoubtable Countess of Rothes was also in attendance, and because the Americans had no royalty of their own, these titled ladies were the focus of the gathering.

"Of course," the English Lady was saying, "I am designing for the future. The next two decades should see a remarkable change in feminine fashion. The modern woman is no longer content to sit at home: she wishes to take her place in the world and requires the clothes to do it. There is a growing movement for the enfranchisement of women in England and the modern Miss does not wish to strap herself into constricting corsets, or to emphasise her figure with bustles, or to hide her legs away in long skirts." There came a rustle of dissension from the traditionalists, but the Lady was a couturier, with shops in Paris and New York, and was thinking ahead for the future.

"Good old Emily Pankhurst!" hooted the Countess. "Do you know we have William T Stead, the famous reformer aboard? Perhaps, he would agree to head our own pressure group: 'The *Titanic* League for Women's Suffrage.'" She was scathing in her derision: not one to hold back on any subject with which she disagreed, and the Chairman hoped, even though his friend was the butt of her jibe, that she would blow this line of conversation out of the water. As a rabid anti-feminist, it was not one he could countenance.

He turned on Mrs Ryerson, knowing her husband to be a steel magnate.

"I have no doubt your husband would be pleased if these ships are a success," he began, hoping to start a whole new line of conversation. "Once they have proven themselves, and the whole world starts to build, his production of steel must surely double within the next ten years."

"I think Arthur might be more happy if they were to sink regularly, then his production would really take off," returned Mrs Ryerson, trying to stay within the general mood.

"Sink!" The Chairman was horrified. "This ship cannot sink. It was built to withstand all horrors the sea can throw into its path... Look!" He hauled the message form, the Captain had given him, out of his pocket and waved it in front of them triumphantly. "This is a message warning of icebergs ahead, and have we reduced speed? Not likely! The *Titanic* will withstand impact even with one of those. In fact, the Captain tells me he will run the ship up to full speed tomorrow, for a trial. I regret, madam, that your husband will never make as much money from building replacements as he will from building the original thing!"

The mercury in the ship's thermometer dropped dramatically as darkness approached, falling ten degrees, in two hours, to just above freezing point. The cold snap was relentless, and the passengers on deck began to drift away; even the most hardy. The *Titanic* began to resemble a ghost ship, driving on into the gathering gloom. Only the blue uniformed Officers on the bridge, and the look-outs in the crow's-nest appeared to inhabit the liner.

The Captain, for the second time that day, was glad of his greatcoat. He slumped down into it, seeking its interior warmth. He was thinking about the ice which was reported to be ahead. It represented no danger in his mind. The deadweight of the *Titanic's* displacement, trolling along at twenty knots, would cut through field ice like a knife through butter. The only danger was from icebergs, or growlers, but because of their bulk, they were easy to spot. This was the busiest sea lane in the world, apart from the English Channel, and hundreds of ships passed along it daily. In his memory, the Captain could not recall one ship colliding with an iceberg to become a fatal casualty of the ocean. Many had suffered damage but none had sunk. The fact that before the discovery of radio waves, numerous ships may have gone down in this way, unable to call for help, or to inform the outside world, did not occur to him. It was inevitable ships would be lost at sea - it was the nature of the element. Their demise would come for other reasons: storms, bad maintenance, poor seamanship, whatever; but he was convinced no such agency would harm his ship. It was, after all, the most modern liner in the world. Yet, in the back of his mind, the stigma of the collision with the *Hawke*, when he commanded the *Olympic,* had burned a deep scar. How would it look if he brought the *Titanic,* his last command, past the Statue Of Liberty and up to the Company Pier in the Hudson River, with her hull plates ripped and her paintwork marred?

"Quartermaster," he barked over his shoulder. "Bring her round two points to port, if you please."

"Aye aye, sir," came the Quartermaster's reply.

The imperceptible change in course, which would take the ship south and west, was not much but, exaggerated by the distance still to travel, would take her well out of trouble if the ice-field did not drift too far south in the meantime. The Captain walked slowly into the chart-room and noted the course-change on the chart. He looked at his watch and noted the time beside the alteration: ten minutes to six. He did a hypothetical plot to see where the new heading would lead him and was satisfied.

When he returned to the bridge, the Second Officer had come on watch.

"Evening, Second," he greeted. He liked the young man, who was a very able sailor and possessed the intelligence to go far.

"Good evening, sir."

"To set your mind at rest, I have had that fellow up before me, today," The Captain announced.

"Who, Mr Peacock, sir? Did he come and make a complaint after all?"

"No... no... not him! The other man, the gambler... Mr... er... ah..." The Captain wrestled with his memory.

"Mr Meredith, sir," advised the Second Officer.

"That's the man," agreed the Captain. "Anyway, I've had him up. Denied everything, of course, very convincing in his innocence, but he did not manage to fool me. Something about those chaps you can spot a mile away. Very plausible in his explanations, but a little contrived. Not much I can do for the other fellow, without a complaint, but I don't think we will be troubled by our Mr Meredith again... well, not on this voyage at any rate."

"We will have to inform the Booking Office, sir. We don't want him back on board again, do we?"

"There doesn't seem to be much point in that. If the man keeps changing his name every trip, I don't see the Booking Office can do much about the situation."

"I will just have to keep my eyes open in future, sir; ground the fellow if he comes on board, before he can do any harm."

"Pity you didn't keep 'em open this time, eh... Second," grumbled the Old Man, without rancour.

"Yes, sir," agreed the Second Officer, happy to accept the rebuke from such an experienced skipper; although the Captain would not have been pleased by the use of his modern terminology.

Tom Pirbright racked his brains to find an excuse which would let him escape from Amy's cloying attendance, so he could meet Sian as he wished. A high proportion of the steerage passengers were Irish, or of Irish descent, and Catholic - it was not the Protestants which were leaving that land. Consequently, there would be no gaiety in the Open Space tonight as Christ's adherents respected the Lord God's proscribed Day of Rest. Amy knew this, from idle talk at the lunch table, and had made plans for Tom's evening without his consent. He would baby-sit all the children, he had been informed, while she and Clara took a turn about the ship for a 'nice' change. Tom was furious but he could see no way round Amy's edict: she was adamant.

"Ya've bin aut every night since we came on board," she had brushed aside his protests, "an' its aah turn naa."

Tom had arranged to meet Sian at eight, before he was aware there would be no steerage dance that night. He had searched in vain during the afternoon, to find her, in order to make other arrangements, and cursed himself for not having discovered where her cabin was. He knew only, her berth was in the stern section, but not exactly where. She seemed to have the knack of disappearing during the day, like a nocturnal animal, and her burrow was impossible to locate. What would she do if he did not arrive at the appointed meeting place? In the absence of any news, would she wait for a while, or go away immediately? Would she think he had decided to stay with his wife and end their burgeoning relationship in a vicious blast of spite? The thought he might not have her tonight, in the pristine Linen Room, provoked a nauseous reaction in the pit of his stomach. He needed her so much now! She had invaded his being like the effects of a drug, the craving constantly demanding to be satisfied, although it must be her who was injected with the seminal cure, not him. The thought he might never be able to touch her again was unbearable, and he sought desperately to break the chains which bound him to Amy and his progeny.

What made his situation even more desperate was the knowledge that Amy was only doing this to demonstrate her independence in a 'what is good for the gander' type demonstration, and that she had no interest in the ship beyond it being the means to spirit her away to a new life. She would probably wander around the gangways for half an hour just to prove what was sauce for him was also sauce for her. That half an hour might make all the difference to his plans for the future, but surely Sian would understand if he could not meet her because of his paternal responsibilities... or would she? One thing was sure, there could be no showdown with Amy on the ship. He could only guess, too well, what her response would be, and knew her tears, and her confused emotions, her heartfelt pleas, would break down any resolve he might carry in his heart. If he was going away to Chicago, with Sian, it could only be on the basis he could slide away unseen, and never have to reappear to face the consequences of what he had done to her. Perhaps this was some sort of sign, he had been sent, to show him the error of his thinking; that no matter how bad the bird in hand might be, the bush might hold more surprises, and heartbreak, than he could imagine. This line of thought did nothing but throw him into deep confusion over what he should do, and he felt a another bout of soul searching coming on. However, try as he might, he could not put Sian out of his mind, and knew that, as long as he remained sane, he must try and find a way to slip out of this unwanted tie with Amy, and go on to meet his destiny.

Declan Reilly shovelled the offending coal into the hungry mouth of the boiler's furnace with overt viciousness. He recognised the black cloud which hung over his head as the beginning of a dark, depressive mood which threatened to engulf him. It was not the work which used him so, but the loss of comfort from the long empty bottle of Irish whisky in his lonely, resting hours. He had run out of booze yesterday and had been without a drink for twenty-four hours.

He hardly knew any of this crew - they had only been signed on eight days ago - and had not seen any of his previous shipmates, being stuck down here in this steel prison for twelve hours a shift. The stewards he approached had been an unco-operative lot; brown-hatters for the most part, and not inclined to help anyone who was not of their ilk, or prepared to join in their unnatural rites. As a Catholic, the very idea of that disgusted him beyond belief. He could find no soul aboard, with a secret cache, who was prepared to share a drop with him. The more he shovelled, the more the memory of creamy-tasting stout and the bite of hard liquor tormented his unfulfilled taste-buds; and the more he shovelled to try and relieve his frustration. If he wore himself out, he would fall asleep without enduring the recriminations his deprived body heaped upon him for not bringing a bigger supply, or for consuming it too fast at the outset of the voyage. If only time would spirit by more rapidly to offer some hope of imminent relief, he would be a happy man, but between the four iron walls that held him here and the narrow confines of his bunk, it seemed like time had stopped altogether. He no longer had a cushion of contemplation to help the hours pass by - he had used up all his thoughts - and his actions became more and more zombified; labour without hope being the expectation of the common man in this generation.

Lorna Wainwright was almost back to her happy, cheerful self; the portents of doom just a fading memory. She had taken great comfort from, and been uplifted, by the Divine Service the Captain had conducted. He was the ideal man to take it too, with his fatherly, almost Godlike demeanour; reading out the prayers in his sonorous tones; a refreshing change from the cream-puff vicars who were the norm in her local parish church. He gave the distinct impression that their lives, and their spiritual welfare, were in very capable hands, which negated most of her fears. She wished Jonathan could see the error of his ways, and embrace Christianity, so he might benefit from the comfort exuded by the Lord. Then Jonathan was an island to himself; unperturbable in his own little world.

Molly had insisted on taking tea with Lorna again that afternoon, in the stateroom next door. Lorna could see she was the one who needed consoling now, and was glad to repay the succour Molly had given her, in her hour of need. The two women were becoming firm friends, and it was to Lorna's great regret they would only have these few short days together, until their lives must surely go their separate ways. Tomorrow she had determined to lay on the tea, in her cabin, as she did not wish to become beholden, or a burden, to her recent acquaintance. It seemed to be true that the Lord moved in mysterious ways, uniting people through adversity, and assuaging their fears through His understanding of the nature of man.

From seven to seven thirty, three separate messages came in from the Leyland Liner *Californian*, some miles ahead. Their wireless operator reported the sighting of three large icebergs moving to the south, at Lat 42 3'N, Long 49 9'W. It appeared that the Captain's assessment had been right, the ice field was drifting in the strong current. Actually, if all the warnings they had received that day had been plotted on the chart, in conjunction with each other, instead of being treated in such a cavalier fashion, a very different picture might have emerged. There was an ice field, seventy-eight miles long, directly in the *Titanic's* path.

Harold Bride took the messages to the bridge and handed them to the Second Officer. He in turn passed them on to the Sixth Officer, his watchmate, to mark on the chart, waited for his report, and then promptly forgot all about them; he had other concerns. Bride returned to the Marconi Room, where Jack Phillips was becoming agitated. There was so much work to get out and Cape Race was still not in range; putting it down to weather conditions, which he could not understand as the night was so clear. Perhaps Newfoundland was shrouded in fog, blanking off the radio waves? He could not know that the slight change in course, which the Captain had made, was taking them south, away from the shore station. They would be in range soon enough.

David Peacock took his wife to dinner at seven thirty sharp. The First Class Dining-Room was packed, and they were still a curiosity, although their moment of unsought notoriety was beginning to pass. Other snippets of gossip were already claiming the interest of the other passengers - so-and-so had been seen on deck with so-and-so, and guess who had been seen coming out of whose stateroom last night! The scene was incomparable. Starched white cloths covered the tables as an appropriate backdrop to the gleaming silverware, which flashed and sparkled in the harsh, electric light. The reflected rays, from the jewels of the privileged, flashed and scintillated across the room, added to by the incandescence of the light bulbs in the ornate, moulded ceiling, and the gleam from the stained glass windows, gave the room an appearance of a fairy castle, which one would only expect to see in a Disney film today. The tables were, for the most part, laid for six, with neatly arranged cutlery and folded serviettes standing up proudly, although David had managed to secure a table for four, which no other passengers shared, by the timely handing of a large tip to the Chief Steward before dinner on the first night. Because of their second-honeymoon status, David and Molly had wanted to be alone, and now, in their present condition, on display through no fault of their own, it was working to their advantage. David unfolded his napkin and spread it on his lap. He handed the menu to Molly. Their Table-Steward hovered nearby.

"What would you like me to order you, my love?" he asked with concern. The choice was difficult. The starters were: Hors d'oeuvre Varies, Oysters, Consommé Olga or Cream of Barley soup. The fish course was Salmon Mouseline with Cucumber sauce, followed by Filet Mignons Lili, Sauté of Chicken Lyonnaise and Vegetable Marrow Farcie. Then there was lamb with mint sauce, roasted duckling and apple sauce, and sirloin of beef, all offered with a selection of succulent vegetables.

"I'll have the Consommé, the salmon and the duck," Molly decided after a delay. David was not that interested in food.

"Make that for two," he told the Steward who was busy writing down the order on his pad.

"Vegetables, Madam... Sir?" the Steward queried.

"Something of everything... with Parmentier potatoes?" David raised his eyebrows and looked at his wife. Molly nodded, and the Steward went on his way.

"David, what are you going to do about this man and the money you lost?" Molly inquired while they waited for the Steward to return. "You haven't said."

"No," he agreed. What indeed was he going to do about the money, and Lucas Meredith? He had more or less decided he must search the gambler's stateroom while he was out - from the layout of the cabin he had seen last night, there could not possibly be too many places to conceal a cheque - and looked for such an opportunity. He had to find the cheque, and destroy it; then Meredith could do about it what he liked, even attempt to take it out on David's nose if he felt he was big enough. David did not know Lucas was almost under house arrest, and confined to his cabin, and such an occasion would be unlikely to arise, because the gambler had no intention of renewing his acquaintance with a locked storage cupboard, which had been his fate several times before on previous voyages - not all Captains were as moderate as this one.

"I don't know," David told her, "I have not decided yet. One thing is for certain, I have no intention of letting the man get away with his evil scheme."

"Why do you not take the nice officer's advice, and report the matter to the Captain," suggested Molly, with the best of intentions. "Surely, it is not too late for that?"

"No," said David decisively. "There are several days to go before we dock in New York. Something will turn up, you'll see: it always does in a just world. Anyway, I am sure the Captain has much more important matters on his plate, like running this great ship... I am more than sure he will not want to be bothered by such a trifle." Molly saw, then, he would not be moved and began to fear, all over again, for his safety. Her picture of Lucas Meredith was generated by the writings of Conan Doyle, and other popular novelists of the day, in which the villain was always depicted as a dark and dangerous man, which in Meredith's case, could not have been further from the truth. However, at the time, Molly had no way of knowing that.

Further conversation was prevented by the return of the Steward with the soup.

—

"Shall I call the Wine-Steward, Sir?" he wanted to know, and David nodded his obstinate head.

Tom Pirbright had decided he would have to act at dinner-time. He felt it was the only chance he might get to save the situation. He could hardly walk up to Sian, in full sight of Amy, so had left his plans fluid to suit any situation which could occur. His only problem was that Sian might not turn up in the Dining-Room, but she did, right on cue, with her father on her arm, and took up her place on the other side of the room. Once again, she hardly glanced at Tom, while he cast longing looks in her direction. He was, by now, besotted.

He tried hard to follow the aimless wanderings of Amy's and Clara's minds, but found he could not concentrate. He ran his eyes over his wife's gross body, and began to try and hate her for the need to indulge in subterfuge she had thrust upon him. It proved not to be difficult, and the howling children, who would not shut up, were earning themselves the same fate. Amy had been so fresh and clean once, and full of life like Sian, but now she was degenerating into a blowsy hag in front of his eyes. There was no longer any need for comparison: Amy could not hold a candle to his new-found love. This unappealing domestic scene was no longer a necessary part of his life: he knew what he must do!

Sometime later, when he had screwed up his courage, he pushed his plate away.

"S'cuse me, gels," he told the women, "I gotta see me mate."

"Whot fur?" challenged Amy.

"Well, I was gonna meet 'im tanight, but I can't naa, kin I... not if ya wants me ta look arter the bleedin' kids?"

"It won't do ya any 'arm," began Amy, "ya 'ave bin aut every night since... "

"I ain't givin' ya a bleedin' argument, am I?... Sa don't give me one, alright? I'll look arter the poxy kids fur ya, but I gotta tell me mate I can't make it. I can't leave 'im standing aut in the bleedin' cold all night, if I ain't coming, kin I?" Tom had gone for the overkill, explaining everything, so Amy would not be suspicious. Without further word, he rose from the table and crossed the room. He stopped at Sian's table but did not address her; it was to her father he directed his words. Sudden alarm appeared in Sian's green eyes but he shot her a faint smile to comfort her.

"Allo, Mick," he began, and the Liverpudlian stared up at him with no recognition in his eyes. "Haa ya doin', mate?" Tom was shocked. Sian's father seemed to have deteriorated since he came on board. He looked old, even though he could not have been above his middle-forties. His complexion was grey, and great bags had puffed up under his eyes. The broken blood-vessels in his thin-skinned cheeks told their own story.

"What do you want?" Mick demanded. "Who are you?" Obviously, he had not been allowed his daily ration - because it was Sunday, perhaps? - and was not happy with the side effects of his temperance.

"It's me, ya mate, from va ovver night," Tom told him, but Mick was not impressed.

"Bugger orf, can't you see I'm eatin' me dinner," was all he grunted, and turned away from Tom's searching eyes. Tom looked at Sian instead.

"Can't make eight: see ya at ten," he muttered out of the corner of his mouth, hoping the other passengers at the table would think it was part of the rebuttal to his summary treatment at the hands of Mick. Sian raised her eyebrows quizzically, but Tom shook his head almost imperceptibly.

"I'll see ya later, ven." His voice was directed at Mick but his eyes were on Sian, and she gave a tiny nod in answer. She understood: and Tom walked away with a grateful heart.

It was not until eight-forty that the Second Officer checked the thermometer on the starboard wing bridge. The mercury inside had fallen below thirty two degrees, and he realised the sea down below must be close to freezing. His immediate concern was the ship's fresh water supply, housed in tanks, at the bottom of the ship, abaft the engine room. He hurried back to the bridge and called the engine room on the phone. He spoke to the Second Engineer.

"Can you send someone to check on the fresh water tanks? We're at freezing-point up here, so God knows what it is like down there! We can't have our passengers inconvenienced, now can we?"

"I'll send someone along right away," came the answer through the hand-piece. They chatted for a few moments about the performance of the ship.

"How is it going down there?" the Second Officer inquired.

"Like a well-oiled clock: it's a beautiful job," said the Second Engineer proudly. Neither, like members of a conspiracy, mentioned the fire in the forward coal bunker: on the Chairman's command it was a taboo subject.

"Keep her going then. I'm already looking forward to a break in New York," encouraged the Second Officer. It had been all go since the 9th of April, when he first came aboard.

What they would never know would undoubtedly hurt them both. Metallurgy was not an exact science as yet and the steel which had been used in the *Titanic's* construction was flawed with impurities. As the temperature dropped further and further, and the frigid metal contracted, causing the outer skin of steel plates to tighten on their frames, the hull would become more and more brittle, like an eggshell, ready to crack catastrophically if the wrong type of stress, like a blow from a giant teaspoon, were untimely applied. That particular moment was not far away!

The Captain looked at his watch for the umpteenth time that day: it seemed he was always pressed for time. It was eight fifty-five.

The Weidners had hosted a dinner party in his honour in the à la carte Restaurant - they had sailed with him previously and were old friends. The Sayers were there along with Mr and Mrs William Carter, wealthy Philadelphians, and Major Archibald Butt, military aide to President Taft and a very close friend of Theodore Roosevelt. He was a man after the Captain's heart, experienced, genuine, and with something relevant to say about the world, and who could indulge in a conversation without promoting himself or his business, as the others were wont to do all too often. Much as he would have liked to stay in congenial company, the Captain told his hosts, his routine was already in danger of being disturbed and that would not do at all. Having made his excuses, he slipped away, leaving the Weidners, and their guests, to enjoy the rest of the evening, after saying he would see them all the next day. He made his way along to the bridge.

In truth, he had become rather tired of socialising, and suffering bores - his stockpile of small talk had almost run out over the years - but it was required of a Captain, at the time, as part of his duties. An unsociable Captain could not compete in the booking stakes with a gregarious one, and many Captains had their fans who would follow them from ship to ship.

"Everything alright, Second?" he inquired as he gained the bridge, and the Second Officer, inspired by the Engineer, replied, "Yes, sir, the ship is running like clockwork."

"Let us just hope we have a sound spring," commented the Captain, but the officer dared not query the remark in case the Old Man was feeling testy.

"It is getting very chilly out there, sir, so I have asked the crew to keep an eye on the fresh water reserves."

"Good man... Have we received any more ice warnings?"

"Yes sir, at about seven thirty, while you were at dinner. The steamer *Californian* reported seeing three icebergs to her south. I got the Sixth to plot them on the chart. They are well out of the way, sir, so I didn't see the need to bother you or reduce speed."

"Hmmmph," grunted the Captain. "Visibility is pretty good! I don't think there is any chance of an iceberg creeping up on us, is there, Second?"

"None at all, sir," concurred the officer.

"Well, make sure the look-outs are awake, just in case. Ah well, Second, I'm off to bed. If you are in any doubt, wake me... I shall not be far away."

"Yes, sir, goodnight, sir."

"Goodnight," uttered the Captain as he turned away.

The Second Officer considered the Captain's words for a few minutes. It was the practice to continue at full speed, in these conditions, until an iceberg was sighted and then decide what evasive action might be necessary if danger threatened. The sea was so vast, and ships and bergs so small, it was highly unlikely the two would be on a collision course at any time. The big bergs had broken off the pack-ice hundreds of miles to the north and would be well decayed by now, in these latitudes and at this time of the year, where warm and cold current fought for supremacy. Besides, the eyes in the crows-nest were the keenest on board and should be able to give ample warning if anything untoward might be coming up. To enforce the Captain's command - even competent eyes might tire or be distracted - he called out to the Sixth Officer.

"Tell the look-outs to keep their eyes open for small ice and growlers, will you... and tell them to pass it on when they are relieved."

"Yes sir," came the reply. They were the only precautionary measures he would take.

He stood and looked out of the bridge windows and felt good. He, unlike many officers, enjoyed every moment when on watch. The concept that he was in sole command of the liner's destiny made him pretentious, and filled up the gap in his being which hungered for power and acclaim. One day, and not too far in the future, he hoped, he would be in sole command at all times, his own master, responsible only to the Board of Trade, and the Company's Directors, for his actions while at sea. It was his cherished ambition. He did not look forward to the watch changing at ten pm, when he would be relieved.

By eight-forty, the wireless room had picked up the elusive Cape Race and the transmission of passengers' messages had begun at last, almost frantically. Jack Phillips told the shore station they were likely to be up all night, and geared himself up for a long session. Harold Bride retired to take a short nap; he would be required when Jack's fingers were beginning to tire, and mistakes were likely to start being made. Phillips would call him, the senior operator said. Thus it was when the next warning came in, it would be overlooked, and never taken to the bridge.

The signal was from the *Mesaba,* warning of heavy pack ice and numerous icebergs from Lat 42 N to 41 25'N; Long 49 W to 50 30'W. It should have rung alarm bells in anybody's mind. Phillips wrote it down faithfully enough and put it to one side, with every intention of delivering it to the bridge, but like everyone else under pressure, would leave it until he had time. His first responsibility was to his employers, the British Marconi Company, and the money that was about to be made from these cablegrams could well justify his continuing employment on this comfortable ship. The Assistant Purser distracted him, just then, arriving with a fresh batch of message forms.

"Where do you want these?" he asked, and went to put them down on the desk. Phillips snatched them off him petulantly.

"Give 'em here," the operator demurred. "We can't have them getting mixed up with the ones I have already sent: we won't know where we are," and he carefully placed them on the bottom of the pile, awaiting transmission. The distraction was enough. After he had sent his next message, he placed the flimsy on top of the ice warning, and then another and another. When he had a little pile to the side, he picked them up and stuck them on his spike, so the charges could be worked out when he was not so harassed. The ice-warning would remain there, unseen by anyone, ever again.

At ten o'clock, the next watch, under the control of the First Officer, came on duty. The Second Officer, with a last look forward, reluctantly went off to his bed. Up in the crows-nest, the look-outs were changed. Fred Fleet and Reginald Lee braced themselves for a cold vigil.

"The bridge says keep a good eye out for small ice an' growlers," one of the relieved men told them just before he scooted down below.

"Tell 'em to save us some cocoa, mates," Fleet called out after the departing men.

"Keep a good high hout!" grumbled Lee. "Hit's halright fur them heffing hoficers, they're hall tucked hup on the warm bridge. Hit's cold enough hup here to freeze yer highs hin their sockets."

"Aaah, you just don't know when you're well off," joked Fleet. "Just be grateful you and me get all the good jobs round here." Reginald Lee uttered another profanity.

It seemed to poor Tom he had waited interminably. He owned no watch with which to check the time, and cursed his over-enthusiastic compulsion to arrive early. It must surely be past the appointed hour by now, and Sian was late or she was not coming. Tom began to wonder if she had mistaken his message, and yet he recalled how she had nodded her head in acquiescence.

He had been dead right about Amy. She had returned to the cabin within half an hour, nauseatingly cheerful, and he had been forced to stand her company for longer than he would have liked. She chattered on unendingly, and he had better things to do. She had even encouraged him to go to bed for once, insinuating he might be rewarded, but he could not stand the thought of that now. The air had appeared to perk up her sexual appetite at a most inappropriate time.

"C'mon Tom, gi' us a cuddle," she had said and he knew it was time to go.

"Naw. I gotta take a turn rand ve deck; vis bleedin' stale air is doin' me ead in."

"You gorn mad or sumfink! It's bleedin' freezing aut vere," contested Amy.

"Naw, I ain't mad: I jist need some air, vat's all."

"C'mon Tom, I want ya ta come ta bed," she insisted, with a fraudulent, girlish voice which sickened him - he did not like to see her degrading herself.

"I ain't gonna be long, ya'll jist 'ave ta keep it warm fur me," he told her, knowing he had no intention of returning while she was still awake.

"Ya better not, or ya won't git nuffink," she warned.

Now, as he stood here, he was beginning to regret the decision. Maybe, it would have been best to have abandoned Sian tonight and had a last fling with his wife. But then, he told himself, Sian might have come if he had not, and he could have lost out on her bounty. Panic set in. Had she realised he meant her to meet him here, as arranged, despite the delay? Was she waiting for him somewhere else? What could he do? Then he had a very dicey situation on his hands. If he went looking for her, she could turn up while he was gone, and thinking he had not come, might go away in high dudgeon. If he stayed where he was and she was waiting elsewhere, things might end in the same way, to his detriment. Why was life turning out to be so difficult all of a sudden?

While he was pondering, Sian appeared like a wraith from the companionway, and flitted across the deck towards him.

"Where ya bin?" he demanded, "I bin goin' aut of me brain."

"Im sorry, loove, but me dah ain't been very well. I arra put 'im to bed," she explained.

"I fought ya weren't comin'," he told her disconsolately.

"Warra bout you? I thought yer 'ad changed yer mind, like."

"Naw, not me," he assured her. "Ve old gel wanted ta go fur a bleedin' walk. I 'ad ta look arter ve kids. I didn't fink ya would mind, 'cos it might be ve last time I do it, see."

"No, I don't mind," she said quietly. "Ave yer told hur yet... abou-rus, like... that yer comin' wit me." Tom was horrified.

"Not likely," he protested, "she'll go bleedin' spare. Naw, I ain't gonna tell 'er. I'll jist 'ave ta do a runner, vat's all."

"That isn't very fur," Sian advised him.

"Fair... vat's rich!" he exploded. "Ya turn me life upside darn, and naa ya want me ta be fair. Well, I ain't tellin' 'er. Ya don't know wot she's like: she'll tear me bleedin' 'air aut." The idea of him in that condition seemed to amuse her, and she burst out laughing. Tom was not amused: his cheap, thin coat made no real attempt to keep out the cold, and he could think of warmer places.

"Anyhow, wot we gonna do naa?"

"Worra yer mean?" Sian replied through her giggles.

"Well, we can't stay 'ere, can we... I mean." He cast his eyes around the empty Open Space. "Vere ain't a lotta life up 'ere, is vere?"

"Well, we can't go down stairs yet: it's too early! Thur'll be too many people about," she cautioned.

"Naw. It's too bleedin' cold. Ve'll all've gorn ta bed."

"The snotty passengers, maybe, but the Stewards will still be about. We better wait fur a bit, like... Lerrus go fur a walk," she suggested.

"Ya must be bleedin' mad," he told her. "If we gonna 'ave to stay 'ere, we'll do it my way. Come 'ere, gel, gi's a cuddle."

By ten thirty, the sea temperature was down to 31 F. Tom Pirbright was right: most of the passengers had retired for the night, to find warm cabins, and staterooms, if not to sleep. The decks were deserted by even the most hardy travellers. In the Cafés and Restaurant, a few parties were still in full swing, as was the Palm Court Orchestra, but even at these affairs the ladies were beginning to pull shawls more snugly around their shoulders, and look to their menfolk for an early withdrawal. A few souls inhabited the First Class Lounge, and the Smoking and Writing Rooms, but not in organised groups: only those insomniacs with nothing better to do. A quiet Sunday was almost over, and all looked forward to a better day tomorrow, with milder weather and superior distractions.

Forty miles ahead, the Leyland Liner *Californian* encountered a sea of ice blocking her forward progress. Her Captain, Stanley Lord, decided it was madness to attempt a passage in the dark and decided to stop for the night. He instructed his wireless operator, Cyril Evans, to send out yet another warning, knowing the *Titanic* was coming along behind, to her and any other ships in the area. Being the

Californian's sole operator, that poor man had suffered an overlong day, having been on duty from seven that morning until the present time: not for him the luxury of a relief! He would send his message, be rebuffed, and retire to bed, sorely aggrieved; turning off his equipment in the process, very effectively cutting off the *Californian's* ears.

In the *Titanic's* Marconi Room, Jack Phillips was still wading through the seemingly endless pile of messages. He would not have minded if all of it had been meaningful, commercial traffic, but most of it was domestic twaddle, sent by rich travellers with nothing better to do, to unconcerned recipients, who never bothered to answer. Still, whatever the text, the messages were his bread and butter, and he sent them all in order of arrival now, regardless of the contents. He was in the middle of one such piece of nonsense - some bigwig wanting his personal railway car sent to meet him at New York - when suddenly his earphones hummed and whanged loudly, almost blasting his eardrums. He snatched off the headphones irritatedly: the sender was obviously very close. He broke off from Cape Race in disgust, his transmission ruined, and tapped out a ferocious reply, with angry, agitated fingers:

"Shut up, keep out, I am busy. You are jamming my signal. I am working Cape Race." The incoming signal died - not a word of it having been recorded - and he replaced his headset to call the shore station again.

Declan could not face his bunk, tired as he was, at the end of his shift. In his sorry state of complete sobriety, he had become claustrophobic, and needed some fresh air to ease the throbbing skull-ache which had descended on him in the last hour or so. Before the day when migraine was first diagnosed, headaches were headaches, and this one was threatening to crush his brain. He could not even raise a cheerful smile, or be bothered to joke with his replacement, Leading Stoker Williams.

"How much longer is dis f-hooking voyage goin' to last?" he muttered ungraciously, and Williams replied happily, "Think of the money, boyo," as he always did. There was only one thing Declan wanted the money to buy him, a case of bourbon, and the devil take the Master at Arms when he brought it on board. That started him thinking about drinking again and he had to hurry topside, in an attempt to leave the memory behind. Using the crew's companionway, he came out onto the well deck to find a clear, crisp night on display, with an array of stars twinkling in the dark canopy of the heavens up above his head. It was the first time he had been up on deck since the ship left Belfast.

He started when he saw a grotesque shadow hugging a wall nearby, and then relaxed as he realised it was a young couple cuddling close to keep out the chill. He wore only his filthy boiler suit, and the frozen air slammed against the insides of his lungs as he breathed, but he felt no pain because of the sudden change of environment from humid heat to harsh, dry cold. His alcohol-starved system was beyond physical hurt, his body already stretched on the rack of excessive toil, and his brain had switched off to save his senses from further distress. He walked over to the rail, and looked down into the black sea; lost in thoughts of his home, in Ireland, and the comforts of Mulligan's Bar.

Close by, Tom watched the stoker go by, from where Sian had dragged him reluctantly, to take the air, and hated the man for invading their private world. They had talked and made tentative plans, between the kisses which were designed to keep them warm, but which were ineffective beyond stirring Tom's desire.

"Shall us ga darn," he pleaded, "an' see if we can git in vat linen room. It's late, an' everyone should be in bed by naa. I'll catch me bleedin' deaf if we 'as ta stay up 'ere much longa." Sian was in teasing mood.

"I'm sure it's all yer want me fur," she rebuked him. "Yer can't wait to get me downstairs, like!"

"Yua gotta fink of it as a dance of anover sort," he told her, "but whiff better movements an' lots more fun."

"Come on, then: I suppose yer won't be 'appy till yer've whorus out."

Up in the crows-nest, Fred Fleet blew on his fingers and stamped his feet. The hundred minutes since he came on watch, at ten, had passed slowly and had been totally unremarkable. It was much better to be fully occupied in these conditions - the mind did not notice the pain so much - and he could not remember the last time he had been so cold. Still, in another twenty minutes, Lee and he would be relieved and could go below to find a steaming cup of cocoa to warm them up before they went in search of their bunks. Fortunately, some other poor bugger would have to do the graveyard shift! Twelve to two was always the worst: it was an unnatural time to be about.

He looked ahead, through eyes slitted against the chilling breeze under his woollen hat, and saw a patch of pearly mist some distance ahead, directly in the *Titanic's* path.

"What's that, Reg?" he asked his shipmate, pointing ahead with a lift of his chin.

"Hit looks like 'aze ta me," ventured Lee. Fleet watched for a moment as the ship sailed on, and then panic gripped the pit of his stomach with icy hands. The patch of fume was too localised: all gathered in one place, and surely that could not be right? Before he could speak, Reginald Lee had voiced Fleet's sudden fears from beside him.

"Cor blimey! Hit's hay bleedin' hiceberg: coming straight hat hus." They had no way of making sure, apart from waiting for the berg to materialise: the look-out's binoculars had been misplaced before they left Southampton, and no one seemed to care.

Fleet waited another few seconds, and then rang the warning bell three times to alert the bridge. He snatched up the connecting phone and waited for a reply. The Sixth Officer, the junior on the watch, took his time answering.

"What can you see?" he asked.

"Iceberg, sir, dead ahead." The officer peered out of the bridge window, and the refractive glass gave him no such sight.

"Are you sure?" he asked unhurriedly. "I can't see anything."

"Course I'm sure," Fleet bellowed down the phone, his discipline curtailed by the fright. "That's what I'm up 'ere for, init?"

"What's the range?" asked the Sixth Officer, pedantic to the end.

"I dunno, it's hard to say: maybe a thousand yards." The Sixth Officer replaced the phone and called across to his superior.

"Look-outs report an iceberg, directly ahead of the bow, at about a thousand yards," he stated solemnly, and galvanised the First Officer into instantaneous action. He was an experienced officer and responded immediately. He stepped up to the Engine Room telegraph and rang 'All Stop', waiting for the repeater, down below, to register the command before ramming the indicating lever into the 'Full Astern' position.

"Quartermaster," he barked over his shoulder. "Wheel hard-a-starboard, man, and do it... NOW!" He rushed forward to peer out of the bridge window. The enormous iceberg was taking shape ahead, gathering up its bulk out of a cloud of rising vapour which shepherded it along. It looked very close already. He felt the forward run of the ship being checked by the massive drag of the reversing propellers, and knew, with a catch in his throat as he drew in a great gulp of breath, it would never stop in time. His seasoned eyes watched the bow for any movement, but the massive vessel drove on, into the night, heading straight at the approaching berg. His heart was pounding in his chest; his brain cringing in trepidation of what was to come. It seemed, then, that time went into slow-motion as he waited for the vessel to respond. He gauged the narrowing distance with a dread which fixed his mind in a hypnotic trance; denying access to any other thought.

Yet, as he watched, the impossible began to happen. The lumbering prow gave a point or two to port. At first he could not believe it, but then he had to, as the ship slowly veered away from the obstacle in her path.

"Get round... get round, my beauty!" he shouted at the top of his voice, encouraging her to pay off, unmindful of who might be listening. Then, in his abject terror, he railed, unreasonably, at the growler blocking their path. "Get your filthy carcass away from my ship." At long last the way began to come off the ship and she shivered slightly as the screws found better purchase in the flat sea. The First Officer knew, the slower she went, the quicker she would respond to the helm, and he shouted encouragement. "Come on, me beauty!... You can do it!... Come on!... Get yourself round!" It was as if the *Titanic* listened to his entreaties, and started to come around by the head, more and more, as the gap closed; turning her elegant lines away from the wall of ice, rushing down upon her. It was going to be close, the First Officer could tell, as the iceberg came abeam of the starboard bow, and he closed his eyes, after he had gauged just how far it was away, or seemed to be. He knew that only a small proportion of the berg was above the surface; the bulk of it hidden under the dark water below. While its ragged, decaying sides might miss the ship altogether, the jagged crests of the inverted mountain could slice their way through the liner's hull as if it were the feeble tin-plate of a sardine can; leaving her core exposed to the unforgiving ocean. He did not know how long he held his breath, with his eyes tight shut, before he dared to look, but when nothing came, no ripping, gouging sound of terminal damage, he flicked his eyes open again. The growler was gone from his view and he swung his head to the right to see it passing by, barely fifty feet away from the side of the ship. It towered over the *Titanic*, rising above the height of the superstructure; its sheer, overhanging cliff threatening her menacingly. It seemed to the First Officer that the Almighty must be playing games with them, for as it passed, a chunk fell off, depositing tons of ice onto the well deck with a resounding crash, so close a call was it. The caprices of the wind and tide had cut a half circle out of the ice, on the side of the decomposing berg, and it was through this the *Titanic* sailed; not drawing enough water to be affected by the preponderance below.

To the First Officer's immense relief, the iceberg was rapidly passing down the ship's side without snagging the fragile plates of her hull. Then the impossible happened, and he nearly missed the strange occurrence, because it came from a totally unexpected direction. There came an incredible sound, like the whoosh of escaping steam, and the great ship shuddered and rocked, as if she had been kicked in the side by a colossal boot. As he looked around to see the source of this noise, and new development, his unbelieving eyes beheld a pillar of spume rise up on the other side of the ship, opposite from the berg, as tall as the funnels, and forward of the bridge on the port side. The breeze blew some of it away, and it coated the vessel with fine spray, as if it had just passed though a squall, while the remainder fell back into the ocean like an extinguished font. The First Officer was struck dumb with amazement, and remained rooted to the spot for a interminable time.

No one would ever know how the explosion occurred, and very few on board would even learn about it. The resolute fire, in the forward coal bunker of No 5 Boiler Room, had never succumbed to the efforts which threatened its life. It had burned steadily on, gathering energy, although it never reached the sides where it might have been detected by its heat through the bulkhead. It produced, as it burned, flammable coal-gas, which rose to the top of the compartment, seeking escape. In a purpose-built gasometer, it would have been given room to expand as the drum rose when the pressure built up, but in its confined predicament, it compressed more and more into an untenable space, becoming a time-bomb just waiting to go off.

It can never be certain how it was ignited, or what lit the fuse that set it off. Maybe, the smouldering fire reached a big pocket of oxygen, which allowed a momentary flame, or the braking motion of the ship shifted the coal to release a small reservoir of the life giving vapour. Whatever it was, and however it happened, the bomb blew up with uncontainable force, to hurl its destructive power at constraints which should have been immovable, but were not, to the everlasting detriment of this fine ship. The cataclysmic blast took the line of least resistance: through the steel-jacketed hull, and the bulkhead door, where the metal had been pinned by welding. Rivets flew as the seams popped; zigzag cracks winged across the brittle, outer skin in all directions, at lightening speed; hinges opened out like metal flowers; locking-bars snapped like cast-iron rods; and the coal bunker's door flew across the Boiler Room. In a split second, the fragile, imperfect steel of the hull collapsed in a shower of fragments and a thirty foot hole appeared in the side of the ship, well below the water-line. The hungry, icy sea rushed in, seeking the warm, dry interior of the *Titanic*. It was all over in the wink of a eye, and the once proud ship, lay mortally wounded from a completely unexpected quarter. The rush from millions of tons of pressurised water killed the fire in an instant - where the crew had failed - and washed the jet black fuel out of its path like a powerful cleaning-hose, spraying away particles of unwanted dirt...

Leading Stoker Taff Williams never had a chance. He was dead before concussion burst his eardrums. He was shovelling away unconcerned when the explosion occurred, but never heard it. As the coal bunker door, freed of its metal fetters, flew across the Boiler Room, it picked him up and crushed him against the open furnace doors, popping him open like an egg sac which had splattered on the floor. Even before his juices could run down the heavy metal plate, embedded in the fire-box wall, the gore had been washed away by the cleansing flood pouring in...

The Second Engineer was in Boiler Room No 6, nearest to the bow, when the warning sign lit up on the boiler indicator. He gave the order to shut all dampers, cutting off the flow of air to the fires, when he heard a sound like a huge gun firing close by. The ship rocked as if recoiling from the discharge. A second later, he and his companion, Leading Stoker Frederick Barrett, were drenched by a jet of water, squirting at them through the open coal bunker door. The jet became a gush and then a deluge. The appalling noise, and the sudden shock of the freezing water, was more than enough to send them scuttling through the short passage to Boiler Room No 5. A churning maelstrom of water was cascading into that compartment, and the Engineer knew the hull had been breached.

"Get those fires raked out!" he shouted at Leading Stoker Barrett, and fled astern, towards the Engine Room...

The stokers in Boiler Room No 4 heard what sounded like a clap of thunder, which they knew could not be right, down here, in the bowels of the ship. To a man, they knew what such a noise could mean, and by the time Barrett had recovered his composure enough to issue the Second Engineer's order, his men were gone, clambering up the escape ladders to the safety of E Deck above them...

Declan Reilly had seen it all happen from the well-deck. He had idly watched the iceberg coming up, and had seen the ship beginning to turn away. It started to concern him that the officers were cutting it pretty fine, but then he respected them for their knowledge and experience, believing they knew what they were doing and would protect the liner; no ship he had been on had ever collided with anything before. Even so he held his breath as the berg came abeam and passed on its way. He marvelled at the blue-ice wall: so close, he felt he might even reach out and touch it. When he looked up, he saw how the iceberg overhung the ship, above his head, he was instantly afraid. It was just as well he took such a precaution, as he spotted the block of ice snap off the unstable rim above and come crashing down towards him. He dived for the cover of the companionway, but it was a close run thing, being stung by fragments of sharp-edged ice, on his back and legs, which showered everywhere when it broke up on contact with the solid deck, before he reached a safe haven. He had barely stopped in the entrance of the stairwell, to look back and utter, "F-hookin' hill!" when he saw the plume of water rise up from the sea alongside the ship, on the far side, and heard a muffled thump as the *Titanic* shied away from the venting detonation. He guessed, in a instant, what had occurred, and paused only to cross himself hurriedly, muttering, "Holy Mary, Mudder of God, have morcy onus all!" before he dived below...

The Second Officer stirred in his bunk as the *Titanic* bucked but his dulled senses did not register alarm. His sailor's perception told him the ship was slowing down, and he might have been more interested in this disquieting motion if sleep was not trying to claim his tired body. If he was needed, he would be called, he decided, and turned over to find fresh comfort and warmth...

It came as nothing more than a slight annoyance to Jonathan Wainwright, reading a book while Lorna slept. He lost his place in the text when the bed on which he lay danced with what he would put down, at the time, to a power surge; an extra heave of the engines. Later, when he learnt the official line, he would be confused. He had felt nothing more than that heave; no sense of shock, no prolonged reverberation which felt like one heavy object crashing into another, or ferocious abrading as they ground together. Discerning nothing unusual in all this, he returned to his book. The first inkling he had, that something was definitely wrong, was when the engines stopped dead a few minutes later...

David Peacock was in bed, but was not tired, and sleep eluded him. With nothing else to do, he watched Molly's eyes moving as she dreamed and hoped it was not anxiety which caused the darting motions beneath the tightly stretched skin. She had not said much to him today on the subject of his gambling, as if she had managed to cleanse her soul of troubles, and lost the need to remonstrate with him over what he should or should not do. All day he had looked for Lucas Meredith, and had not seen the gambler about; not at meal-times, or in the Smoking Room, as if the man had decided to avoid him, and stick to the comfortable cabin. Now, David planned how he could winkle the cardsharp out, in the time he had left, by some subterfuge which would allow him to search Meredith's stateroom. He felt the ship begin to slow down and then shudder, but had no opinion as to what it might be. He returned to his scheming...

Lucas Meredith was a well travelled man with a wealth of experience on the ocean. He looked up from the book he had almost finished and wondered what had caused the shudder he had felt through his chair. He remembered a vessel on which he sailed once, throwing a propeller under full steam, and thought this movement to be not unlike that experience. Whatever it was, it would most likely be a problem for the Captain, which would keep him occupied for some time, and as far as Lucas was concerned, after his run-in today, it could not have happened to a nicer chap! However, he saw it as a chance to venture out from these depressing four walls for a bit, without being noticed, and stood up, dropping the book on the chair he had vacated. He stripped off his ostentatious smoking-jacket, which was not the best wear for keeping a low profile, and searched out his anonymous black overcoat...

The Chairman had only just turned in when he sensed the unnatural motion of the ship. He lay and wondered for a moment what might be the reason. Why should she stop in the middle of the night?... Unless... and he remembered the ice warning, in the message from the *Baltic,* which he still had, in his coat pocket, from earlier in the day. Could it be? No... he had felt no rumbling scrape as he might have expected in such circumstances, and yet when the crump came, transmitted by the frame, his alarm accelerated into sudden fright. Still, his orderly mind tried to justify the digression from the ship's normal motion. He would have expected to hear a ripping sound, like a gigantic fingernail being drawn along the side of the liner, but it had been nothing like that. He could not rest now, with all this going on in his mind, so there was nothing else to be done but get up again and try and ascertain the cause of this unsatisfactory disturbance...

Thomas Andrews was working on his blueprint, noting suggested modifications he had just worked out on his scribbling-pad. He was in tune with the ship to the extent that he knew every squeak, hum and moan emanating from the mechanical systems, as if the continuous resonance she emitted to his senses was one of his bio-rhythms, locked up deep inside him. He lifted his head and listened as he detected the gigantic propeller shafts, in the well of the ship, winding down, to momentarily stop, and then wind up again. He guessed at once something was desperately wrong. It was not normal practice, and dangerous to the bearings because of the strain, to go from 'Full Ahead' to 'Full Astern' so dramatically, and no Captain would order it unless he was trying to avoid something solid, like a concrete quay or another ship. Andrews detected the drag in the ship's motion as her massive screws ran up to full speed in reverse, and a few moments later had his fears realised when the jolt of the explosion was transmitted to his feet through the deck. Yet, still he did not move: frozen in mid-motion like a diorama, pen clutched in hand, while he listened and waited for further developments. He did not want to know what had happened to the vessel; whether she was damaged or how badly. It could only reflect on the work he had done, on the design, and the changes he had been forced to make, against his better judgement, because he would not stand up to his biggest customer, the Board of Directors of the White Star Line. If the *Titanic* was in danger, he was not yet prepared to face up to it, and he remained where he was, unable to move...

Tom Pirbright, spliced into Sian, was the only one unconcerned by the turn of events. It seemed to him, with this glorious connection finally made, that the tremor was the earth moving beneath him; a just reward for his efforts, engendered by Sian's obvious love for him, and his for her; irrevocably consummated. It would not be until much later on, when a growing commotion in the gangway outside reached his ears, and was assimilated in the aftermath of their passion, that he would perceive something was not quite right with his little world...

The Captain was on the bridge within a few minutes. Some innate sailor's sense had warned him that all was not well with his ship, and roused him instantly from a deep slumber. The explosion occurred when he was discarding his pyjamas and hurriedly pulling on his uniform. The First Officer was on the phone to the Engine Room when he arrived.

"What is going on? Why are we stopping?" he demanded. The First Officer could only point to the window and mutter, "Iceberg, sir."

The Captain looked out, over the starboard side, and saw the growler disappearing astern; its bulk untroubled by the boiling wake, thrown up by the churning screws as they back pedalled turbulently.

"Did we hit it?" the Captain wanted to know, and the First Officer shook his head, trying to absorb two voices at once, one in each ear.

"No, sir."

"What then?"

"We've suffered an explosion... down below," the officer reported.

"How... Where?"

"I don't know yet, sir; I'm trying to find out." The Captain's mind raced, trying to cover all possible connotations.

"Is the hull broached? Are we taking in water?" he interrogated, and the First Officer nodded, obviously distressed.

"As far as I know, sir."

"Have you closed the watertight doors?"

"No sir, not yet. I am waiting for a damage report."

"Do it NOW, Mister," roared the Captain, snatching the receiver off the shocked officer; who then hurried over to pull the lever which would electrically seal the hull into isolated segments.

"Who is that down there? This is the Captain speaking," the Old Man bellowed into the mouthpiece, hardly needing the instrument to transmit his voice through the several decks which separated them. "What is happening? What has exploded? What is going on down there?" The questions came out like rapid fire from an automatic gun.

"It's the Second Engineer, sir. I'm not sure what's happened. The Chief is taking a decko now, sir. We are badly holed and taking on water, as far as I can see... It's a bit difficult, sir, we... "

"Where are we holed?" the Captain cut in.

"Port side sir, in No 5 or 6 Boiler Rooms, sir... I think!" came back the disembodied voice, and the Captain knew the worst in a flash.

"It's that damned forward coal bunker," he mused aloud and then returned to the conversation. "Tell the Chief to report as soon as he knows wh... " the Captain had begun until a much better idea struck him. "Never mind," he shouted and slammed down the receiver.

When he turned back to face the world, he was everything a commander should be: cool, calm, rationally controlled. He spotted the junior officer of the watch, standing idly by.

"Sixth... find Mr Andrews, the designer; give him my compliments, and ask him to come up to the bridge."

"Yessir!" called out the young man, as he took off.

"Hold on, Sixth... I am not finished yet," the Captain checked him. "After that, rouse all the officers. Tell them to get dressed and to assemble here, on the bridge. Now, off you go quietly: we don't want to start a panic, now, do we? Say nothing to anyone, not even the officers. Do you understand?"

"Yessir."

"Oh... and Sixth... take your time. I don't need one of my officers nursing a broken leg, or the like, not just at this moment."

"Yes, sir. No, sir." It was a much calmer young man who set off from the bridge on his appointed tasks: his courage bolstered up by his respected superior's austere words. The First Officer had returned to his side.

"Ring engines 'All Stop' if you please," the Captain ordered, just as the Chairman appeared in his sight, much to his chagrin, and he sighed a deep sigh of resentment. It was the one person he did not need interfering in the present crisis.

"What is happening? Why have we stopped? Have we hit that iceberg?" the Chairman wanted to know when he arrived at the Captain's side. He could not fail to notice the berg, as big as a cathedral, as it went away directly in the *Titanic's* wake.

"No we have not," the Captain said angrily, not prepared to accept the responsibility of another collision. "It appears we have suffered an internal explosion. I've sent for Andrews: to get his view of any possible damage."

"An explosion! What sort of explosion?" questioned the Chairman.

"I am not quite sure yet. I am expecting a report on the matter, from the Chief. It would seem the seat of the explosion was No 5 or 6... " The Captain's voiced faded as his composure cracked. "It's that forrard coal bunker, dammit: I know it is. Why wouldn't you let us deal with it properly in Belfast? How the devil did I let you talk me into sailing with that fire alight?"

"Poppycock. You know nothing concrete: you just said as much." Then the Chairman's expression became inscrutably bland, and the Captain thought he must have gone into some sort of trance. "There has been no explosion. We have hit an iceberg," the Chairman announced quietly, and the Captain felt he had guessed the man's condition correctly.

"No, sir: you don't understand. We have suffered an explosion in one of the forward Boiler Rooms," he corrected, as if he were speaking to a child, only to be met by the Chairman's implacable stare.

"No, Captain. It is you who do not understand. I said, there has been no explosion on board. The ship has hit an iceberg. Now do you comprehend?" the Chairman insisted. The Captain fell in suddenly, and knew there was nothing wrong with the man. It was just like him to say what he had, and the Captain did not like what had been proposed.

"We cannot say that: the truth will out," he protested.

"No, it will not, not if we do not allow it to," he was told for his trouble. "It cannot... must not come out, we had an explosion on board. That's bad for business - very bad for business - and I will not allow it. You will put it out that we have struck an iceberg."

"But, sir, you could never get away with that! If there's an inquiry... "

"An inquiry! Why should there be an inquiry when no other ship is involved? We've been bashed by an iceberg, man, that is all we have to say. The ship is not going to sink, is it?" The Chairman had lost his poise now, and his voice rose as his control vanished.

"Well no, sir, I think not, with only one compartment breached. Five or six would have to be flooded before we were in any danger," the Captain had to admit. "I've seen to it that the watertight doors are closed."

"Who is to know, then? We can say what we like! I... " The Chairman dried up as Thomas Andrews appeared. The designer, finally galvanised into action by his conscientiousness, had met the Sixth Officer on his way up to the bridge, saving valuable time.

"What has happened? Why have we stopped?" Andrews asked the universal question.

The Captain opened his mouth to speak, and had framed the word 'we' with his lips, when the Chairman spoke for him, as if not trusting what he would say.

"We've struck an iceberg," the Chairman conveyed to the designer. Andrews would never be told the truth, and would not see the damage close at hand. He was not a threat to the Chairman's conspiracy.

"I would like you to take a look," said the Captain, seizing control. "I would value your professional assessment of our condition."

"Of course... Is it bad, do you know?"

"Not too bad, I shouldn't think. It was only a glancing blow, you see," the Chairman butted in, much to the Captain's annoyance. He should not be doing this: trying to upstage a Commander and take control.

The Chairman placed his hand on Andrews' shoulder and turned him away. He knew Andrews very well, and could take such liberties.

"We need a quick report, Thomas," he submitted. If the designer could be fooled then anyone could, and the Chairman knew it. He would not let the Line, his very life, be castigated for negligence. The iceberg was so far behind now, no one could say with certainty which side of the ship it had passed, well, no one who could be called upon to give evidence, that was! "We won't be able to see much until we have her dry-docked, of course, but we want to keep this as low key as possible; for both our Company's sakes... what! Not a word to anyone about what you find... eh... old chap... except the Captain and myself, naturally."

"No, of course not," Andrews remonstrated hotly as if he had just been insulted. He looked towards the Captain, pulling away from the Chairman's cloying grasp. "I'll take a look down below, right away. Which way is it, this hole?"

"Forward in the bow," the Captain informed him and did not like the way the designer grimaced, as if he knew something everyone else did not. The time was just on midnight as Andrews set off.

"You see, his report will say we struck an iceberg, and everything will be alright," concluded the Chairman gleefully. "He designed this ship, and no one is likely to argue with him!" The Captain wished, just then, the Chairman might be washed out of the hole, in the side of the ship, for his effrontery; but then realised no one could be that fortunate on an unlucky day!

THE LAST DAY

Thomas Andrews returned to the bridge sooner than expected, with the downcast appearance of a very worried man. His shoulders had stooped a little, and his eyes were sad and soulful. At first, during the swift inspection, his brain would not acknowledge what those eyes had seen, and yet he had come to accept the inevitable because of its implications for the passengers and crew.

"Well, Thomas?" the Chairman bullied him as soon as he appeared. The Captain would have liked to take the designer to one side, to receive his report in private, as he was still Master of this ship, but the Chairman had proved to be unshakeable in his tenacity, and hung on where he was, at the hub of events, successfully blocking every recommendation the Captain put to him, about his having better things to do, with a straight, defensive bat.

"Well... " began Andrews nervously. "Things appear to be worse - much worse than we anticipated."

"Come on, man: spit it out!" encouraged the Captain. "It surely cannot be that bad."

"Bad!" echoed the designer. "You don't know the half... "

"Well, Thomas, you've got to tell us sometime: it might as well be now."

Exasperation was creeping into the Chairman's tone.

Andrews gathered himself up to his full height, and delivered his report in an even, mechanical voice.

"We are holed in compartments five and six, on the port side, at a point roughly between hull frames No's 58 - 60. At the rate the water is rising, it suggests we have a rather large hole, say twenty or more feet across, through which the sea is pouring unabated. Although the major damage is to Compartment No 6, we are also taking on water in No 5 - fortunately at a lesser rate but still rapidly enough to cause me great concern."

"What about the pumps? Surely they can contain such a leak?" the Chairman queried expectantly. Andrews continued brutally.

"The water level in No 6 has risen twenty eight feet in the last twenty minutes. At that rate, the pumps would have no chance of holding the level. In No 5 Compartment, they may hold for a while, until... " Andrews' voice died away.

"Until what, man?" demanded the Captain.

"Until what?... Until what?" echoed the Chairman. Andrews sighed.

"Until the water in No 6 reaches the top and overflows into No 5... and No 7, naturally." The Captain was speechless, but the Chairman spoke for him.

"What do you mean... overflows? Those compartments are watertight, are they not?"

"Yes," Andrews agreed wearily, "but only up as far as E Deck. When the water reaches the top, it will flow over into Compartment No 5, and then No 4, and so on, like the ornamental fountain in your garden, sir."

"Mr Andrews: what are you saying?" The Captain sought to clarify the unspecific information; to know the worst. Andrews looked at him sorrowfully.

"I am saying the ship will undoubtedly sink. The bow will fill up and the weight of water will drag her down by the head. Then the sea will gradually permeate the rest of the hull." The Chairman exploded in a gale of rage.

"Sink! This ship cannot sink... it is unsinkable!" he roared.

"No, I do not think anyone at Harland's ever claimed that," Andrews told him in a quiet way.

"You did!... You did! You assured my Board it was unsinkable, when you foisted your revolutionary designs on us!"

"No!" stated Andrews a little more forcibly. "I think you can look towards the press for that epithet... The press and your own publicity machine."

"How dare you!" bawled the Chairman. "Lord Pirrie himself assured me the design would render it unsinkable." Andrews shook his head dolefully.

"I think you will find what Lord Pirrie said was: 'that it is the safest ship afloat'. None of our ships have ever suffered this sort of iceberg damage before. I do not think anyone foresaw these circumstances."

"What! You stand there and tell me your design was duff: unworkable at the first hitch. After all the millions we have spent at Harland's, I expected better than that. I mean, none of this was mooted when you took over from the dreadful man Carlisle. My Board was told we had the best man available, and now you have the audacity to inform me this ship was never what you claimed it to be... unsinkable... invincible." Andrews had no immediate answer: he had not expected to be attacked on the personal level.

It was the Captain who came to his rescue.

"Gentlemen... please! This is not the time for grievances: it cannot alter our situation." He turned his attention to the designer. "Mr Andrews: you say the ship will surely sink because of the water we are taking on. If we get under way and proceed at best speed, will this not lessen the intake of water to a point where the pumps can manage better, or at least give us more time to make a landfall or the like." Andrews shook his head again.

"I think not. Forward way will only help to push the bow down deeper in a shorter time; for the sea will be forced into the hull, by the pressure, at a faster rate. Nor can I see any advantage in going astern, as in time, when the bow begins to sink, the screws will lift out of the water." The Captain was forced to accept the death sentence on his ship.

"How long have we got?" he asked deflatedly, as if all the wind had gone out of his sails. Andrews thought for a moment.

"I don't know... it is hard to say. An hour and a half... two hours at the most: I could not definitely say the ship has longer to live than that."

"Thank you, Mr Andrews, for your honesty at this difficult time," the Captain told him sympathetically, sensitive to his melancholy mood, understanding what the admission had done to his pride.

"This is all nice and comty," the Chairman shouted hysterically. "The bloody ship is sinking... doesn't anyone realise that. Captain... I would like a word in your cabin, in private."

"Not now, sir," sighed the Captain. "There is much to do and I..."

"It was not a request, Captain. I want a word in your day cabin... now!" The Chairman turned and walked away, leaving the two men staring after him in shocked surprise. It was some few moments before a very angry, and agitated, Captain made a move to follow him.

"You and Mr Andrews do not seem to realise, there is a lot more at stake here than just losing a ship," the Chairman said, having calmed down somewhat in the intervening few minutes. "It is not a question only of how a ship was lost, but also why it was lost! But then I do not need to tell you that, do I?"

"I think you need to tell me everything, sir: because nothing you are saying makes any sense, to me, at least," the Captain replied.

"What we are talking about, here, is damage to the Line, don't you see? The ship in itself is no great loss - it is well insured - but the Line is not, and we must limit the damage to it as best we can. To be blunt, we both know there are not enough lifeboats to carry everyone away, and over half the passengers and crew must stay behind to take what chance they can. What we must do is make sure the right people survive."

"If any good can come from this, let us hope it might be the Board of Trade will review their out-dated regulations concerning lifeboats," mused the Captain, and the Chairman tutted in exasperation.

"I don't think you have understood a word of what I've said," he upbraided his employee. "Do I really have to spell it out for you, Captain, word by word?" The Captain nodded at him.

"I wish you would, sir, as what you say is going completely over my head. Forgive me if I do not understand, but then I am only a simple sailor and not familiar with business practice, like yourself." The Chairman sighed deeply.

"This is not about the ship: it is about people. People sue, not ships, and the richer they are, and the better reason they have, the more they will look to receive. There are a great number of people on board, and if they all sue for damages over this, it could well see the end of the White Star Line, and I am not going to stand here and see that happen. In the first place, we will maintain our story that an iceberg was responsible for the damage to the ship - and you will put out distress calls to that effect. The greater the number of influential passengers who survive this night, the better it will be for the Line as they will have no plausible cause to claim over an unavoidable accident. The others - the steerage and the crew - are of no account and cannot damage us with legal action they cannot afford. You will ensure the First and Second Class passengers are put into the boats, and the rest will have to take their chance." It was the Captain's turn to explode.

"You cannot do that, sir: it is downright inhuman. The lore of the sea says, 'women and children' first and then 'every man for himself' after that. We cannot play God, and pick and choose who shall die and who shall not."

"Very noble!" remarked the Chairman casually. "And my lore says it shall be done my way in the best interests of the Company, who has fed us both, very well, for a number of years. You will give out we are sinking through iceberg damage, and you will lock all barriers on the ship to prevent the steerage passengers, and the crew, from swamping the lifeboats and leaving before the other passengers are away."

"Over my dead body, sir," snarled the Captain, and the Chairman replied, "It might well come to that." The two men faced each other toe to toe; at loggerheads, as they had been so many times before; unable to accept the other's right to authority. The Chairman was the first to recover.

"Captain, let us be reasonable. By the morning we will both be dead - for we shall be the last two to leave - so what difference does it make to us what happens when we are gone. There is a million and a half pounds invested in this ship alone, and if our insurance does not pay out, because of our negligence in sailing with a fire on board, and the passengers sue, for the same reason, it could cost several million more... God knows how much. Then there is a further million and a half invested in the *Britannia,* still on the slipway - and who will want to sail in that after we have proved to be... shall we say... neglectful in our responsibilities."

"And whose fault is that?" accused the Captain. "If only I had not listened to you... I should never have done... at Belfast, this would never have happened."

"Captain... Captain! It is too late to apportion blame now, and history will never know whose fault it was if you will play it my way. J P Morgan, whose Trust owns International Mercantile Marine, has been disturbed at our results of late, and has been talking about selling off the Company for some time. Such a disaster as this, through negligence, with the cost likely to bring us to the point of bankruptcy, would likely push him over the edge, and persuade him to disband the Line completely, selling it off piecemeal to the highest bidder. Dead or alive I could not stomach that! My own father built up this Line, and brought it to what you see today, with my own poor efforts contributing, over the last few years, since his death, and I, for one, cannot go to my grave thinking our once proud ships had been sold off to be abused by squalid, profit-grabbing owners! The White Star Line has nurtured me, and been my whole life, as it has done and been for you, and we cannot let it end in this way because of some silly mistake I made in Belfast, when I only had the Company's best interests at heart. Would you want my eternal rest spoilt, and on your conscience, because I made a mistake? I know you only too well, Captain, and do not think you could do that to any man." It was a beautiful speech, contrived to earn sympathy for him, so he would obtain his own way. The Captain did not speak for some long time. When he did, it was not what the Chairman wanted to hear.

"I'm sorry, sir, I cannot go along with this deception. I am, I hope, a man of honour and integrity, and because of my position, ultimately responsible for this tragedy. Though it might have cost me my command, I should never have allowed you to override me at Queenstown. Therefore, things will be done my way, and I shall tell the truth about what has happened here tonight, and in Belfast. I do not think these people, and the world, deserve to be deceived. Now if you will excuse me, there is much to be done and little time." He turned to go but the Chairman moved in to block his path; a terrible fury raging in his eyes.

"Captain," he began in a curious, high-pitched voice, as if he had screwed up all his courage, and emotion, for this moment. "I am still the Chief Executive of the Line, and your employer. If you will not see things my way, then it is not too late to have you replaced as commander of this ship. The Chief Officer has shown some ambition in that respect, and can be appointed, at very short notice to take your place." The Captain was astounded.

"You cannot do such a thing. I will not stand for it. In any case, none of my officers will gainsay my commands: I am their Captain and they will do what I say."

"I would not be too sure of that," the Chairman told him ruthlessly. "I think I can say I am a better judge of human nature than you. There are many among your officers who would jump at a chance of this command, even if only in her dying hours. It would be a major accomplishment for their future, don't you think, if they could say they had commanded the *Titanic*."

"I thought you said the crew were all going to die," sneered the Captain. "Which of them will have a future?"

"Anyone that I decide," returned the Chairman. "If you will not co-operate with me, I will take command through one of them. I will be the one to decide who leaves this ship, and who does not. A place in a lifeboat will be its own reward. The promise of that, and a dazzling future will be enough to ensure I get my way."

"You are a fiend, Sir!" the Captain shouted at him. "And who do you think will listen to you from among my crew?" If he thought his words would dismay the Chairman, he was wrong.

"I would have thought the Master at Arms might be a good place to start. You would be surprised what the offer of a lifeboat place, a handsome bonus, and the thought of being made Chief of Security for the Line might do for him. Shall you summon him, Captain, or shall I? Shall we put this man's loyalties to the test?" The Captain was very much inclined to do so, but hesitated just a moment too long. It convinced the Chairman he was not sure of his ground. "Well, what shall it be? Will you be there to see your ship go down, as any good Captain should want do, or will you miss it all, locked in your cabin under guard and relieved of your command, at the last moment, like the scapegoat you will become if you force my hand. You and I will not get off this ship, but many of my friends, on board, will. What I tell them before they leave might well colour what history will believe about your particular part in all of this. Believe me, Captain, I know what I should do!" The Captain listened to his tirade and thought the Chairman had truly gone mad: his mind turned by the sudden shock of realising he was going to die. The Captain could face that eventuality much more stoically, but not the idea of disgrace the Chairman had catalogued.

When the Captain spoke, it was quietly, with sage reasoning and good sense; like a father advising a son.

"But sir, can you not see, you will never get away with this. Too many people know about the fire. The truth will out whatever you may try to do. You have no hope of pulling off such duplicity."

"Who knows about the fire but us, a few of the officers, and one or two of the crew? I made sure only a minimum might know in case of such an eventuality. None of those who knows will ever get off this ship in the lifeboats, and if Andrews is right, and we have only two hours before we sink, how many will survive all night in a freezing sea? Not I or you, Captain, for we have seen the day of our heroic deeds." The Chairman had already made plans for those who might survive.

"But, sir," the Captain again tried to talk some sense into this obviously deranged man.

"No buts now, Captain. You are either with me or against me, and if the latter is the case, you already know where that will lead. Dishonour and disgrace await you if you take against me, for that is what I will ensure for you, with my friends' stories of how you behaved at the end; requiring locking up to contain your hysteria and shocking cowardice in the face of adversity. Or if you prefer, you can have your day of posthumous glory as the noble Captain who courageously went down with his ship. Which will it be? Which version of the story will your family want to hear, I wonder?" The Captain went cold as he heard the Chairman's words.

"You give me no real choice, do you, sir? Alright, I will comply with your evil scheme for the sake of my good name, but I warn you; if by a miracle I survive, the whole world shall know what sort of man you are."

"Which is a very long chance I will have to take... You will obey my orders then.?" checked the Chairman.

"I said, I have no choice," the Captain surrendered.

"Good man... good man! As you said earlier, we have things to do. You will return to your bridge and give the order to close off the ship. I want a strict control on who is allowed to reach the boat deck. I shall be there in person, so I would not try getting an informant past me: I shall vet all who leave. Of course, when you put out a distress signal, you will inform the world we have struck an iceberg. You will also give a wrong position as our location. Say ten miles away from our true position." The Captain had decided by now he had truly gone mad and it might be best to humour him.

"But we cannot: it is madness! If we can find a ship to come to our aid, ten miles may make all the difference to the numbers who survive. For those who cannot fit into the lifeboats, it will be their only chance."

"No one is going to find this ship," the Chairman told him coldly. "If she is lost, she will be lost forever, and with her the truth about how we came to meet our end. I still do not think you understand quite what I have said to you, tonight. While I breathe, the world will think this ship was lost by Act of God, and not by anything we have done. When she sinks beneath the waves, the White Star Line's reputation will float to the surface above us, safe for all time. No one will ever know the truth, if I have to kill everyone on board to preserve it. Now do you understand?" he said finally, and the Captain could only mutter disconsolately, "Yes."

"Now we are wasting valuable time with fruitless argument. Captain, you will proceed as I say, for you know the consequences if you do not. It is your own choice, and one that I cannot make for you." The Chairman turned and walked to the door, where he paused and looked back. "Captain, I shall be watching you, and I am not a man to be easily fooled. You do your job as best you can, as I know you will, and keep this ship afloat for as long as you are able. In return I will save as many of the precious passengers as I can, to salve your troubled conscience; I promise you. You are a brave and sensitive man to stick by your principles to the last - I admire you for it - but I must salvage what I can of the Company's reputation, by any means available to me. I hope you will respect me for that, at least! What I do, I do not for my own profit, or gain, but for the thing I love most of all in life! The White Star Line. I shall be proud to die alongside one such as you; a fitting end to my endeavours. If we should survive, by some miracle, I hope you will give me the chance to show you what I can do for you if you keep the Line's good name intact, or I shall see you on the other side, as they say, where you can berate me for evermore, if that is your wish. I have your word, I hope, that you will keep our bargain?" It was then the Captain realised he had been touched by, what he believed to be, this man's sincerity, and wondered if he had not judged him a little too harshly. He was right, after all, when he said he would not gain from his deception and his zealous motives seemed to be genuine.

"You have my word," he heard himself say.

Jack Phillips and Harold Bride were on the point of changing over shift, when the relief pipes on the funnels, close to the radio shack, began to vent steam in a continuous blast, as the boilers were shut down. Although they could hardly hear each other speak, it did not affect their transmissions, as the voice was not involved.

"What's that?" shouted Bride, recently roused from sleep and still mussy. "Why have we stopped?"

"I don't know!" Phillips yelled back. He possessed much more experience of ships than his junior and liked to display his superior knowledge when the chance arose. "Probably engine trouble: one of the boilers sprung a leak perhaps, and they've shut it down to work on it."

"Will we be stopped for long?"

"I don't know! As long as it takes, I suppose, but one thing you can be sure of: there will be no rest for us tonight, me lad. The sort of passengers we've acquired this trip will want the world and his wife to know about this." Before they could appreciate the joke, the door burst open and the Captain stormed in. His face displayed a terrible scowl, and his dark, wild eyes encompassed them both, filling them with apprehension as to what, he thought, they might have done. He had no need to raise his voice: his deep, resonant tone cut right through the sound of venting steam.

"Gentlemen, the ship is going to sink in about two hours' time," he informed them quite calmly, despite his awesome demeanour. Phillips and Bride stared back at him balefully, shocked into silence by the announcement. The Captain continued. "I want you to start transmitting the C.D.Q. distress call for assistance at once. Keep calling and do not stop until I tell you to do so. Is that understood?" Both Phillips and Bride nodded deliberately. The Captain had to get another ship to the *Titanic's* side before she sank: it was imperative! Such a course was the only way he could think of to clear his name and implicate the Chairman in the cause of this disaster and to allow the truth to come out, although he had not yet perceived how it would be possible. If he died out here in the ship, with its fate unobserved, he would never be able to refute what was said about him, and he did not wish to leave disgrace behind him. Killing the Chairman with his bare hands, for holding such a gun to his head, would not have been beyond him at that precise moment. He considered for a moment what he should tell the wireless operators to send, and then decided against taking a chance with his reputation for the sake of his family and grandchildren. He had no doubt the Chairman would do as he had said if he did not get his own way: not being a man to be dismissed lightly. "You will say we have struck an iceberg and are sinking fast. Ask any ship close by to come to our assistance with all speed. Our estimated position is, and write this down - Latitude, 41 degrees 46' minutes North: Longitude, 50 degrees 14 minutes West.

This is, as I have said, an estimated position, and if they cannot find us there, they must come on until they do. I shall attempt to keep our lights burning for as long as I can and shall start firing distress rockets every fifteen minutes." It was as far as he was able to go without risking the Chairman's wrath and calling dishonour down on his head, however unjust that might be. "Keep calling continuously, as our signal will also provide a beacon to draw them in."

"Yes sir, at once, sir," said Phillips, at last able to speak through his consternation. He turned to the set, and with shaking fingers, began to tap out C.Q.D.

"Do you know if there are any ships close at hand?" the Captain asked.

"Yes, sir, I think so, sir. I had a call from someone close at about eleven o'clock," Phillips admitted over his shoulder, raising his voice so the Captain could hear.

"Who was it? How far are they away?" The optimism in the Captain's voice was not matched by Phillips' spirits, which sank as he remembered what he had said through his transmitter.

"I don't know, sir, I'm desperately afraid I brushed them off." He turned back to face the Captain with misery and pain distorting his features. He tried to explain, stumbling wretchedly. "I didn't write anything down... You see, sir, I was working Cape Race... they cut in on me... blasting in my ears, they were... I didn't realise... I told them to clear off the air... I was busy... I... Oh God, what have I done?"

"Can't be helped: you weren't to know," the Captain told him kindly. "Still, if they called you, they must have a wireless. Keep calling until you raise that ship. Tell them to come fast or I cannot imagine what the consequences will be. Find me that ship, wherever she is... tell them to come now."

"Yes, sir," promised Phillips, stung into action by the Captain's words, and his own stricken conscience.

"Blimey," uttered Bride when the Captain had gone. "We're going to sink." His complexion was ashen with fright. "And here was I thinking we were on our way back to Belfast to have the engines fixed." He was staring ahead, as if in a torpor.

"Harold, snap out of it," insisted Phillips. "Get yourself over here. I'm going to need your help: my fingers are burning with transmitting now. What is that new distress signal which has been recently agreed?"

"SOS, I think," muttered Bride.

"Yes, that's the one." Phillips had known all along, and his fingers were fine, but thought it best to keep the youngster occupied, the easier to alleviate his fears.

When they came to put out the new call, it would be the first time such a mayday had been transmitted by a vessel at sea!

As Andrews had predicted, the ship's bow was already sinking into the sea, when the Captain returned to the bridge and confronted his assembled officers.

"What is our status?" he wanted to know, and the Chief Officer gave him a full report. The Chairman lurked irritatingly nearby.

"We are down by the head, sir, as you can see. The squash court is awash and the Mail room is flooded. Water is getting into the holds and the fireman's tunnel is under water. The bow appears to be filling rapidly."

"Have you evacuated the passengers and crew from up forrard?" he demanded.

"No, sir: not yet. The Chairman said..." and the Chief Officer looked nervously in the great man's direction.

"Never mind what the Chairman has said: I am in command here." The Captain blazed, and turned to glance defiantly at the Chief Executive, receiving only a mocking smirk in reply: an unspoken reminder of his predicament. "See that they are brought up onto the well-deck and held there until you have my command to move them. They are, under no circumstances, to be allowed up onto the boat deck until you have my say so. See to it, Chief."

"Aye aye, sir."

"And now, gentlemen, we will go to boat stations," the Captain announced, addressing the other officers. "First, you will take the starboard side and the Fifth will assist you. Second you shall have the port side with the help of the Fourth. I know you have not had any boat drill on this ship but you have all gone through the procedure many times before. Find yourself some able bodied seamen: uncover the boats and have them swung out on the davits, if you please. Loading will commence as soon as the passengers are assembled, and remember, it is women and children first. The men can go when the women are away. Allow one seaman for each boat and no more. There will be no panic, gentlemen: not aboard my ship. I want you all to draw a revolver from the armoury, as you go, and use it only if there is no other choice. Any questions?... No? Off you go." The Captain turned to the Third Officer.

"Go below and find the Chief Engineer. Ask him to keep the lights going for as long as he can: they will provide a beacon for any passing ship we might contact. And then, find the Master at Arms and ask him to come to the bridge." The Captain needed to have the ship's disciplinarian on his side just in case he decided to wreck the Chairman's unholy design.

"Yessir," came the reply, which was smartly overridden by the Chairman's dulcet tones.

"Don't bother with that. I have already detailed the Master at Arms." It appeared the Chairman was keeping one jump ahead. The Captain turned on his protagonist. He managed to keep his temper in check but only just.

"Off you go, Third," he muttered as he ground his teeth together in cold fury. "What do you want me to do, sir?" It was the Sixth Officer asking, feeling put out to think he had not been assigned a task at this important time.

"You will stay on the bridge in case you are needed. Just at this moment, take some glasses out onto the wing and see if you can spot anything... a ship... out there. If you do, let me know and we will call her by lamp. Very shortly, I will want you to organise the distress rockets."

"Yes sir," agreed the Sixth Officer suddenly full of importance, and a little too cheerful, in the circumstances, for the Captain's liking. But then he was so callow and normally irrepressible.

The Captain waited until the young officer had gone. Somehow he held his temper as he addressed the Chairman calculatedly.

"And what have you detailed the Master at Arms to do?" he demanded.

"To keep the steerage passengers in the stern, away from the Boat Deck, of course... as we agreed," the Chairman answered quite innocently.

"When I conceded to your odious bargain, I did not appreciate that you would be sitting on my back, like a monkey, for the whole time the ship has to live," the Captain complained. He could hardly take action to thwart the man's plans if he was constantly under observation.

"In the circumstances, you can hardly blame me for wanting to check," the Chairman told him infuriatingly.

"There is no need to check: I gave you my word. I, at least, am a gentleman and will keep it. There is no need for you to run around anticipating my orders with those of your own. Now, kindly clear my bridge and do what you have to without being under my feet all the time. I do not think there is much more we have to say to each other, do you?" The Chairman grinned wryly.

"You know, Captain, I almost hope you will survive just to see how you would set about making a meal of me! I am sure it would be most innovating. However, I doubt whether either of us will be given the chance to say anything at all, hopefully, and must make peace with our Maker, and each other, as best we can." Surprisingly, the Chairman held out his hand. "If we do not see each other again, I hope you will not think too badly of me. What I do is for the best, and the continuance of the Line. I hope you will see that eventually!" The Captain turned his back then, refusing to take the proffered hand. The Chairman shrugged. "Just as you like," he muttered regretfully, and then his voice changed, to become riven with angry emotion. "We have an agreement, so stay on your bridge and away from the Boat Deck: the officers up there will do as I say. Please recognise the fact, Captain, I have the power to besmirch your name as long as one lifeboat remains on the ship and I will, if I think you are going against me. I certainly would not want you to be remembered in that way, and I do not think you will either by... "

"Get off my bridge before I throw you overboard myself," roared the Captain, and the Chairman departed with alacrity.

Declan Reilly dived down the companionway and tried to get back down to the Boiler Room from whence he had come. He could not get far, being pressed back by the welter of humanity, stokers like himself and grease-monkeys, trying to escape from the water raging below.

"Wha's happenin'?" he shouted to a passing face he knew.

"The ship's holed, an' we're leaking like a sieve," he was told.

"Has annie-body sin Taff?" he called out. "Has annie-body sin Taff Williams?" But no one seemed very interested in socialising just at the moment. They continued to push past him like a herd of frightened horses; jostling and snorting to escape from their apprehension. Declan flattened himself against a bulkhead and hung on for grim death to escape being carried away by the surging throng. He had to wait until almost the entire shift had gone past before he could make further progress.

He came to the ladder above Boiler Room No 5 and looked down into the turbulent maelstrom below. He was surprised how high the water had come in such a short time, and guessed, in an instant, the ship was terminally holed. The water churned around like the action of a whirlpool and it was nearly impossible to tell from which direction it issued, but Declan guessed, in his heart of hearts, where it was emanating from: a large hole, in the hull, adjacent to the forward coal bunker which he had found to be alight when the ship lay at Queenstown. He was one of the few who had seen the iceberg pass by and knew it was on the other side of the ship. What had gone on here, and the explosion he had heard, were not part of anything to do with the growler. He still felt concern for his shipmate, the Leading Stoker, but then realised if Taff had been close to the seat of the explosion, he was either dead, or more likely, would have been the first man out, and was probably enjoying a cup of cocoa in the galley by now. Declan stopped worrying about Williams, and concentrated on what he should do for himself. He decided to go aft, while he still could, and see if there was anything to be done there, or if he was needed. Not many would see things as he would, and perceive that working together for the common good was the best solution in calamitous times.

He would get to the rear of the ship, and up a couple of decks, before the barriers were utilised to keep out the unwanted.

"Whassat?" grumbled Tom as his long wind-down from passion was disrupted by the sound of running feet, and excited voices, in the corridor outside. He had not even noticed the ship had stopped, or the vibration had ceased, and immediately thought the commotion might be something to do with him being here, out of bounds, in Second Class, with a woman who was not his wife; as guilt-stricken adulterers often, unreasonably, do.

"I dunno," declared Sian uninterestedly. "Perhaps yer berra take a luke, like." Cringing with the unpleasant anticipation of undesirable discovery, Tom quickly adjusted his dress and opened the door a crack to peer out into the corridor beyond. What could he say if Amy had set off a manhunt for him, by reporting him missing? Had he overdone the foreplay and prolonged the wonderful act tonight, well overstaying his usual time? He could hardly claim innocence if he were caught in a cupboard with a strange girl! He need not have worried about that overmuch.

A long straggle of people, mainly passengers and stewards, were hurrying past in the general direction of the stern, intent on their own business and taking no notice of him. He turned back to Sian and saw she was fully clothed; nice and respectable once again.

"C'mon, gel. Let's git outa 'ere. Vere's somefink goin' on." They slipped out into the stream and went along with it; nobody seeming to care who they were or where they had come from. Tom caught up with one of the stewards.

" 'Old up, mate. Whas goin' on?" he inquired.

"The ship's 'it an iceberg," said the Steward, apparently unconcerned, for the moment, that he was obviously a steerage passenger.

"Blimey, mate, is it goin' ta sink?" Tom wanted to know.

"I dunno. The Keptin 'as ordered all the passengers to the Boat Deck whiff their life-jackets on. That's all I know."

"Bleedin' 'ell!" ejaculated Tom.

"Me dah," wailed Sian, "Whoras 'appened to me dah?"

"I dunno," grunted Tom, instantly concerned for Amy and the children.

"Will yer come an' 'elp me find me dah?" Sian asked him plaintively.

"I don't know abaut vat," Tom told her as he stopped, incredibly torn between his love and responsibilities. The girl would make up his mind for him.

"Yer tole me yer looved me," she remonstrated. "If yer do, yer will come an' 'elp me find me dah." Her green eyes flashed at him malevolently, daring him to contradict her. "If yer don't, yer better get back to the wife an' kids, like, cos I don't want yer any more." It was enough to decide him.

"C'mon ven, gel: let's go 'ave a look." He took her by the arm and hurried her along with the crowd.

They found Mick in a airless cabin, at the back of the ship, which stank of rank body odour mixed with the sweet bouquet of exhaled alcohol. He was lying on his back, dead to the world, snoring and exuding little grunting noises from between his slobbering, salivating lips.

"Oi," complained Tom, "'e's drunk as a lord."

'"E musta found whur I'd 'idden 'is drink," reflected Sian. "I wunder 'ow 'e did that!"

"Never mind abaut vat! Whatta ya gonna do abaut 'im?"

"Well, we can't leave 'im 'ere, can we, like? We'll 'ave to get 'im up on deck," Sian proposed. Tom put his arm around Mick's shoulders and heaved. He was a big man, Sian's father, and was a deadweight; seeing he was unable to give them any assistance.

"Blimey," moaned Tom. "Es like a bleedin' jumbo. We ain't niver gunna move 'im from 'ere, gel."

"Yer would if it was yer dah," Sian disagreed. "Are yer gonna 'elp me or what?"

"Yas, alright," grumbled Tom and took up the strain once more.

Jonathan Wainwright was still reading when the first soft tap came at the door. He sighed in annoyance and put the interesting article down. Not another interruption, he thought to himself irritatedly. Lorna was asleep on the bed beside him, hair spread out on the pillow, and he did not want her disturbed: it had been hard enough, since they came on this ship, to get her to sleep, although she had improved over the last couple of days. Even so, in his studied way, he would not hurry to answer the door, searching on the floor for his slippers, and adjusting his dressing-gown, until he felt fit to receive whoever was knocking. It was a bit inconsiderate, he decided, for anyone to call at this hour!

As a consequence, another knock, a bit more determined this time, came as he crossed the stateroom. Lorna stirred in her sleep.

"Alright, alright, I'm coming," he muttered under his breath as he reached the door. "Yes, what is it?" he snapped at the white-coated Steward who stood outside.

"Sorry to bother you, sir, but the ship's 'it an iceberg. I am sure it's nothing to worry about, but the Captain wants all the passengers to dress in warm clothes, put on their life jackets and go to the Boat Deck, sir." Jonathan's intestines turned to jelly, and he thought they might slide out of his sphincter unchecked. It was as if he had been punched in the face; his shoulders slumped as his head fell back in abject terror.

"Are we... are we... going... " was all he could say.

"Sink!" the Steward finished for him. "Gawd bless me, no, sir. Hit's only a precaution, I should think... You know what captains are like... hey... sir, like old women at times. He probably finks it's a good time for a boat drill, if I knows the Old Man. Anyhow, this ship can't sink... we all know that." The Steward was quite chirpy as he delivered his message, but nothing he said was any consolation to the wretched Jonathan. "Now I best get on, sir, I've got the others to tell," said the Steward almost regretfully, as if he would have liked to spend the rest of the night chatting idly.

When he had gone, and Jonathan had shut the door, the scientist found he could hardly walk back across the room to the bed, so terrified had he become. Lorna was awake and beginning to sit up in bed as Jonathan wobbled and toppled towards her. Lorna took one look, and her waking, smiling expression changed to one of concern. From the look on her husband's features, she deduced he had been rocked to the core.

"Whatever is wrong, Jonathan?" she asked, and when he replied she could sense the panic in his voice.

"The ship's going to sink... we're all going to drown," he wailed pitifully.

"Nonsense, dear," contested Lorna. "You've been sleep-walking again and have had a bad dream, that's all."

"No... No," he wailed, looking around at the door with horror in his eyes, as if searching for a spectre which threatened to assail him. "The Steward just said... we're to go to the Boat Deck. The ship has hit an iceberg."

"What nonsense," Lorna upbraided him from the security of her new found confidence. "You have imagined it all. Really, Jonathan, you have only just managed to persuade me how silly I have been, and you've begun now!"

"No... no," he echoed in a throttled voice. "The Steward... at the door... he just told me. The ship has hit an iceberg and we're going to sink." There was something about his adamancy which convinced her, and his stricken face was evidence enough for her.

Then a strange thing happened. It was the hitherto irrational Lorna who took control of the situation, in the absence of her petrified husband's capability. She was, at once, cool and collected as she questioned him.

"And what did the Steward say we must do?" Jonathan struggled to remember but it was difficult to recall; his brain had unhinged itself in this sea of troubles, no longer working like the steel trap it once had been.

"We must dress in warm clothing... and then... then go to the Boat Deck... I think he said."

"Was that all?" demanded Lorna.

"Yes, I think so... no, he said we must take our... our life... " He could not say the word.

"Our life-jackets?" queried Lorna. Jonathan thought for a moment.

"Yes... I think that was it."

"Right," stated Lorna assuredly. "We shall do just that. Jonathan, you will get dressed in a jersey and your thickest flannels, while I get the girls up and dressed. Then you will look after them while I get dressed. You can put them into their overcoats, and their life-jackets while you are waiting, and don't forget your own overcoat: it will be quite chilly out there with icebergs about, I shouldn't wonder." She stopped in mid flow. "Oh dear, I wonder if Molly knows about this. I would expect so, but then she is a long way away. Hurry up, Jonathan, we shall have to take care of those children next door, the Peacocks; just in case their mother can't come for them. And we'll have to look after old Nanny as well!" Jonathan was going to be more trouble than she imagined. Instead of following her instructions, he sat on the bed with his head in his hands, moaning and groaning.

"Oh God, how did I ever allow myself to be talked into sailing on this ship. I should have listened to you, Lorna, and got off when we could. You were right! Whatever are we going to do?" Lorna came close, and stroked his hair as if he were a small, frightened boy.

"If we all stick together and you listen to me, we will be alright. I am sure things are not as bad as you think. Come on Jonathan, get yourself dressed," she crooned to calm him, and began to help him shed his dressing gown.

Lorna Wainwright would prove to be, despite her earlier peculiarity, a tower of strength in the time the *Titanic* had left to live. She would certainly not recapture her own inadequacies.

David Peacock, in his First Class stateroom, found out about the trouble in the same way as Jonathan had, from his Cabin Steward, but his reaction was completely different: the news causing his stiff upper lip to click smartly into place.

"Righto," he informed the Steward, "you can leave things with me." He crossed to the bed and tenderly shook his wife awake.

"Molly... Molly, dear, you must wake up." Molly stretched luxuriously, but he could see from her startled eyes, she was not properly orientated. She yawned and asked, "What time is it?"

"It is not morning yet, but it is time to get up," he encouraged. Then she took in his face; solemn and severe before her.

"What is the matter? What is wrong?"

"Nothing to concern your pretty head about," he assured her. He had believed every word the Steward had told him. The ship was in no danger and it was only a zealous Captain taking precautions. After all, the very name *Titanic* spoke volumes in itself: what could do her, of all ships, any harm?

"It seems the ship has had a little bump with an iceberg. Nothing serious the Steward says. The Captain wants us all to dress in warm clothes, put on our life-jackets and go to the Boat Deck."

"Is the ship going to sink?" demanded Molly, startled into wakefulness by the tidings.

"Good Lord no," David assured her, "It's only their way of showing us what good hands we are in. It has happened to me several times on other trips I've taken. It is a matter of them being seen to be doing the right thing while they sort out the troubles. I've no doubt we will be under way and back in bed in half an hour."

"David, what about the children?" the practical Molly remembered.

"Oh they will be alright: Nanny's with them. Heaven help any ship having the audacity to sink under Nanny, what!" He sought to make light of the situation to soothe away any fears she may have. "We must do as the Captain says, my love. Get dressed up warmly and go up to the Boat Deck with your life-jacket, there's a good girl. I'll cut along to Second Class and see to the children, and Nanny of course, if she will allow me. I will join you up there in a few minutes." Molly was easily reassured. David was a world traveller and must know what he was talking about.

In truth, it was the opportunity David had been waiting for and he would seize it with both hands. Meredith must have had the same warning and surely vacated his cabin, long since, as he did not have any constraints on his hands. Who would think to lock a cabin under these circumstances? A better happenstance might never present itself, in the time David had left, and he determined to stop off, on his way to fetch the children, to see if he could find the incriminating cheque. He could only hope the gambler had not been correct when he said it would never be found.

Lucas Meredith had been wandering around the ship for some time. He believed his initial guess was not far out, until he saw the alerted passengers heading for the Boat Deck with their life-jackets on. With his experience to call on, he knew this would not be the case if the liner had merely thrown a screw. A passing steward advised him to retrieve his own life saver, and head for the lifeboats, still playing down the seriousness of the situation to avert panic. It was a precaution, the man told him, and Lucas did not believe a word of it. He had been around ships long enough to know that, with this class of privileged passenger to keep happy, Captains did not call unnecessary boat drill, at this time of night, unless there was a very good reason. Yet, the tingling presentiment that danger threatened could not compare to the thrill of holding a winning hand, and the possibility did not worry him unduly. Despite living through several emergencies, on the ships he had patronised in the past, he had never been shipwrecked - trusting the officers and crew to know their own business best; as he knew his - and was not concerned that anything untoward might occur. For this reason, he did not rush to his cabin for a life-jacket, preferring to stand aloof from the herd and wait until it was all sorted out, saving him the inconvenience of being pushed and pulled about in the throng. There would be time enough to collect what he needed from his stateroom, if the worst came to the worst, while the women and children were being got away in the boats, and the cast iron nerves he had developed to ply his trade kept him completely calm.

So it was he went into the First Class Smoking Room for an undisturbed cheroot and found himself alone with a man he had not seen about before, sitting at a table by himself, staring at the stained-glass windows. Never one to pass over a mark without a closer inspection, whatever the circumstances, Lucas paused beside the table.

"It seems we are having a bit of trouble," he remarked conversationally.

"Yes," the other man replied, not bothering to look up at Lucas or even unfix the rigid stare he was bestowing on the sailing ship, framed in the leaded ties which held the glass in place.

"You, like me, do not seem to exhibit concern, and I, for one, cannot think it might be overly serious. I am sure we will find it nothing but a storm in a teacup," persisted Lucas, determined to elicit some sort of reaction from the man. The reaction he received was not the one he expected. The man, at last, looked up and attached a half hearted gaze to the gambler, but the look in the eyes was still far... far away.

"I, unlike you, know the situation to be very serious indeed, but am unconcerned only because I know there is nothing to be done about it." Thomas Andrews was not in the mood for any sort of small talk.

Lucas was afflicted by a sudden bout of uneasiness. Who was this man and what did he know that Lucas did not?

"Are you sure it's serious? Is the ship going to sink?" he interrogated, and when the man did not reply, added, "How would you know, in any case?"

"Because I helped design the ship," admitted Andrews. "What you see around you is my grand blueprint come to life... Believe me, I know." The panic rose in the gambler's breast as his glands secreted adrenaline into an unprepared blood stream.

"Are you sure?" he queried in a shocked voice, cheroot forgotten and his legs ready to carry him to the Boat Deck with all possible speed.

"The ship has hit an iceberg and is holed: there can be no doubt about it," Andrews uttered wearily. Even though Lucas was set to run away, something held him there; fascinated. He saw in this man something he had never seen before; complete serenity, as if having already accepted an impending fate and come to terms with it, calmly and rationally, finding it no longer held any terrors, or was it the biggest double-bluff he had ever seen? Whatever it was, it was something Lucas could admire: the ultimate poker face.

"If you have known this from the start, why have you not gone to the Boat Deck long since?" Lucas wanted to know, as a student of human nature, and saw something die in the eyes that held him. When Andrews spoke, it was as if Lucas was receiving an unpremeditated confession, and he could do nothing but listen mesmerised, as a priest might be when hearing explicit sexual details from one of his flock, who had strayed.

"There are not enough lifeboats on board to carry everyone away, and I suppose it is all my fault. I should have stood up to the Board when they cut Carlisle's original allocation to the ship... but I did not. I should have insisted on more than twenty although I know the final four collapsibles were only installed as a sop to shut me up. I allowed them to convince me this design was invulnerable, when I knew it was not, because I did not want to be removed from this project, as Carlisle has been when he would not eschew his principles." He looked up at Lucas with supplication in his eyes, as if he needed to explain; to offer justification and be absolved. "You see, I lost sight of my own insignificance, believing myself to have solved all the problems which could occur on any plane and yet I never thought anything like this could happen to my ship." He shook his head in disbelief. "Who would think she would hit an iceberg and need all those lifeboats I did not fight to have installed..."

His voice trailed away as he realised what he was saying to a complete stranger, but then realised it was too late now to withdraw his unburdening. When he continued, his voice had lost its ethereal quality and become matter-of-fact. "So you see, there is only room for half the passengers in the boats. The rest, and the crew, must take their chance in a freezing sea until help comes, from whatever source. I am responsible for their plight, and for all who die, because I did not have the courage to put myself out, when I had the chance, and champion their interest before those of my paymasters. I will have their blood upon my hands, and my conscience is not man enough to bear the responsibility, I'm afraid." He looked at Lucas keenly, and asked, "In those circumstances, do you think I have the right to find a place for myself in the lifeboats; which I did not provide enough of in the first place?"

It was a question Lucas did not feel qualified to answer, though the implications of it, as mooted by the designer, were not lost on him.

"If you are asking me, I would say it is every man's right to look after himself first in a shipwreck situation. In my book, everyone has the same right to life, whatever they have done, and it seems, to me, to be a case of 'the devil take the hindermost', but then I cannot speak for you as I obviously do not have the same high moral standards. If this had occurred on land, I would have shown everyone on board a clean pair of heels, but perceive this cannot be the case here, in the far reaches of the ocean. I would say you have every right to your place in the lifeboats, and urge you to come with me this instant, to the Boat Deck." What Andrews said then would have a profound effect on Lucas Meredith.

"No." The designer denied the argument. "I have no rights. I had my chance in life, a good chance - much better than some - and have been found wanting by my pride. There are many on board who have not had their chance yet, to succeed or fail, and what right have I to take their expectations away from them by usurping their place in the boats, by using my privileged position. Somewhere on board ship, there might be an even greater designer than me, with a more humble attitude, who will someday build a ship which might conquer the ocean. What right have I, who has already failed, to take his chance away by my own selfish desire to live? There are barely enough boats to take the women and children off, and they have no blame to bear, as they go where their husbands and fathers bid them, without choice, so who am I to claim my right and deny them theirs. I must stay here and take God's medicine in whatever unpleasant form it might come." A great weight seemed to have shifted from his shoulders and he held himself erect, in the chair, once more. He looked up at Lucas again.

"And you, sir, must make your own judgement on how you have conducted your life, before you feel you have any rights over the innocent." Then he looked away, back to the sailing ship. "If you have to jump overboard, strike out from the ship and get clear as soon as you can to avoid being trapped in the suction as she goes down. Good luck and God help you," was the last thing Andrews said before he fell into deep melancholia.

Lucas realised he had been dismissed by the man, who obviously did not want to talk any more, and he turned away from him in respect of his wishes. The urgency had gone out of his legs and he no longer felt the need to run away. Perhaps the man was right in what he said, and the stand he had taken was a valid one. What right did anyone have, in an untenable situation, to preserve himself above all others? It was a conundrum with which he would wrestle right up to the moment the ship died. Just now, he decided, he should run with the pack to see what chances might come up, before he could decide whether it was right to take them or not, according to his conscience. He set off for his cabin to find his life preserver. The fraught predicament was beginning to excite him, like an exacting hand of cards.

Declan Reilly had made his way up onto the Boat Deck long before the passengers began to filter up through the Grand Staircase, and the Second Class Entrance at the back of the super-structure. He had circumvented the barriers by working his way round and up from the stern, often passing through the gates just before they were closed. By now, a cordon of seamen, and stewards, under the control of the Master at Arms, had cut off escape to the upper decks, for the Third Class Passengers, out in the open where barriers were not in place, or easy to get around. The Master at Arms was taking his orders from the Chairman quite literally, and any steerage passenger who tried to break through was forced back with violence. These wretched travellers would be held until the last possible moment, and the same system was being employed at the bow, to keep them in at their place in the advantaged queue. It would be a terrible indictment, at the subsequent inquiry, that the class system was allowed to continue even in relation to the boats: those who had paid the most would be the first away.

Declan was not concerned by any of this, or the rights and wrongs: he had merely made his way here as he thought it was where he could do the most good. He had seen the uncontrollable vortex below and knew the ship did not have long to live, and in his Christian way, had come here to offer his services to his fellow man. By his grimy dress, he was instantly recognisable as a member of the crew - among the passengers, for who would clothe themselves like that, other than for a Fancy Dress Ball, which had not been on the entertainment agenda for the day? - and was collared and put to work by the Second Officer, soon after he appeared. The boats were to be lowered by hand and the gear-wheels, which controlled this operation, were stiff and new, and needed several sets of muscles on each to turn them round. Declan, used to riot and civil disobedience in his homeland, as well as the transgressions of parochialism, religious and political strife, and abject self interest, was totally surprised by the discipline and stoicism of the assembling passengers, mainly English, of whom he had no good opinion. They seemed to be treating the whole affair as a merry lark, milling about chatting and exchanging trivial conversation in the carnival atmosphere, as if this inconvenience was the price to pay for having just enjoyed a jolly picnic.

Declan decided he would never properly understand human nature, especially that of his country's usurper, the upper-crust Englishman who made up the Landlord class, and concentrated on the work he had been given, so as to put such thoughts from his head. Instead, he remembered his empty bottle of Bushmills, and licked his lips at the memory. Soon, if his luck changed, he might be offered brandy, or such like, after his ordeal, for it was what the victims of shipwreck were always given in recompense for their suffering, the subsequent celebratory drink, but had to admit it was a hell of a way to find a drink to quench his raging thirst.

Lorna waited as long as she dared, in the corridor outside, reluctant to interfere, but nobody came for the children in the cabin next door. She had superintended her own family's preparations and then told them to wait while she went to take care of the Peacock children. When the nanny opened the door to her urgent knock, Lorna could see the children were already well attended to. They had been dressed in several layers of their warmest clothes, and their Life-jackets were firmly tied in place.

"No, there is no sign of Master... Mister David," Nanny said in answer to Lorna's opening question. "Then I would expect him to make sure Mrs Peacock was safe before he would worry about the children." Then, she either read something into Lorna's expression, which disturbed her, or she did not wish her former charge to be badly thought of, for she added by way of explanation: "He knows they're in good hands, you see."

"Of course, Nanny," Lorna agreed. "I am sure he thinks that!"

"Perhaps Mister David is unable to come," proposed Nanny as an alternative. "The Steward was not very specific about what has happened, and he might have been prevented from coming or is injured in some way."

"God forbid!" commented Lorna, though the possibility was not one she could deny with any conviction. "Well, my family are ready to go to the Boat Deck. Perhaps, to save Mr and Mrs Peacock's concern, I could take the children along with me. I am sure we will find them up there, safe and sound."

"Excuse me, Mrs Wainwright, but I have been looking after young Peacocks for over forty years, and the children will be quite safe with me!" exclaimed Nanny huffily, and at any other time, Lorna might have thought her words quite funny, as if she were claiming to be some sort of female gamekeeper.

"I did not mean I thought you were not capable of such a task, Nanny," Lorna said hastily in consolation. "I meant only, it might be best if we all went up together. We might well meet Mr Peacock on the way. I am sure he will be coming for the children as soon as he is able."

"Well, yes... alright," agreed the nanny dubiously, perhaps realising it was no time to sit on any high horses. "John, Rebecca, come along," she said sternly and gathered the children into her arms protectively.

David was getting very annoyed. He had rifled the stateroom quite efficiently, for an amateur, and had seen no sign of the elusive cheque. The longer it went on, and the more frustrated he became, the more careless he was in the search. He had looked in all the obvious places; in chest-of-drawers and bedside cabinet; in the pages of the magazines on the occasional table and between the leaves of the book he found on the chair; among the collection of menus and other shipboard bumf which Meredith was obviously collecting as souvenirs: all to no avail. He turned his attention to the wardrobe then, and checked through all the hanging garments he could see, although there were very few to choose from. He went back over them again, when he came up empty-handed, to see if there were any hidden pockets he might have missed. If he had been a little more experienced, he might have noticed the Life-jackets still in place, above the wardrobe, but was too intent on his quest to take in that sort of detail.

Greatly perplexed, he stood in the centre of the room and looked around. Where else could one hide a cheque? He crossed to the bed and stripped back the bedclothes untidily, checking under the pillows and down inside the covers, leaving them in disarray when he discovered nothing. It was then he noticed the suitcase, carelessly left on the floor beside the wardrobe. He retrieved it and laid it on the bed. He expected it to be quite packed with clothes, because Meredith had nothing much out in use, and because of the considerable weight, but found only underclothes, two white shirts and a couples of ties inside when he had snapped off the catches and opened the lid. There was still no sign of the cheque when he fumbled through the clothes over-anxiously. It was a puzzle in more ways than one. Meredith had definitely said the cheque was well hidden, in the cabin, where no one would find it, and what better place to secrete it than his suitcase, among the folded apparel, although he was careless to have left it unlocked? Then, the suitcase was too heavy for the clothes it contained, being only of cardboard construction; cheap and shoddy, its exterior finish battered and scratched with misuse. David thought, at once, something was not quite right here. He tipped the contents out onto the floor and laid the case back down on the bed; the better to examine the interior. No secret compartment was immediately obvious; the shabby lining did not appear to have been tampered with; the case looking quite ordinary to the untrained eye. He tapped the bottom without effect and then looked at it very closely. Was it thicker than it appeared to be? He put a hand on both sides, in and out, and tried to feel the depth of it but it was impossible to tell accurately. Then he tried the same device on the lid, and could definitely feel the contours of his probing fingers through the thin, reinforced paper, which was not the effect he had felt through the bottom layer. He became convinced the case was fitted with a false base, but how to get into it was still a mystery. He turned it over and examined it carefully, failing to notice that some of the rivets, which held it together, were slotted to take a screwdriver. If only he had a knife, the fortified, bonded wood-pulp would not have been a problem. A paper knife would do at a pinch but he could not remember seeing one about, and wondered what sort of sharp implements a man like Meredith would keep about him while travelling: a pair of scissors to trim his moustache perhaps? David's spirits sank when he recalled Meredith was a clean-shaven man.

There was nothing for it but to take the case back to his own stateroom where he was sure he would find several sharp instruments, to utilise, among Molly's effects. A clean shaven man... that was it! Meredith must possess a cut-throat razor and it would be ideal for the job in hand. He was already moving in search of it, when a whiplashing voice stopped him dead in his tracks.

"What the deuce do you think you are doing, Peacock?" David swung around guiltily. Lucas Meredith was just inside the door, wearing a very troubled expression which David took for one of extreme hostility. He had been so intent on finding his cheque he had not heard the gambler enter the stateroom. Cold fear flushed up his unprepared system. He had never considered being caught, and had no idea what sort of man Meredith was. As far as David was aware, he might be capable of anything.

At twelve-fifteen, when the news reached them, the ship's orchestra, off their own bat, began to play some lively ragtime numbers in the First Class Lounge. Later they would move up to the Boat Deck, with their life-jackets on, and continue to play, by the port entrance to the Grand Staircase, in an effort to keep the growing number of passengers assembling there, cool and calm for the coming ordeal. By twelve-thirty, the seamen's quarters, and the steerage berths on E Deck, forty-eight feet above the keel, forward of the ruptured coal bunker, were flooded. The bow was beginning to sink beneath the flat sea as Andrews had predicted.

Over the next two hours, several ships would hear the *Titanic's* urgent, bleating cries and prepare, at differing times, to come to her assistance, though most were too distant to make contact before the stricken liner sank. The nearest ship, the *Californian,* would not hear her. Her Captain was asleep in the chart-room and the wireless operator had already retired after a sixteen-hour shift, to fall into an exhausted sleep. The Third Officer was the only other man on board interested enough to listen to the wireless that night, but his knowledge of Morse Code was rudimentary and he did not understand the distress signal. Whether or not this ship was ever close enough to see the *Titanic,* or render early assistance, would never be successfully established, as the liner was not at the position she claimed to be. Captain Lord would deny, to his dying day, that she ever was.

The saddest recipient of the distress call was her own sister-ship, the *Olympic*, five-hundred miles to the east, and heading for England after her own successful voyage to and from America. Her officers would huddle on the bridge, devastated by the knowledge they were powerless to help.

Tom, with a Herculean effort, and not a little help from Sian, finally managed to drag the inert Mick up to the open deck, aft of the superstructure, only to run into the cordon of seamen and stewards the Master at Arms had established, to keep the lowly from forcing their way up to the Boat Deck.

"You can't go past 'ere," a steward told him, as Tom tried to force his way through; desperate to be relieved of his cumbersome burden.

"Why not?" he demanded.

"Cos the Captain says," he was told. "None of you lot is to go any further until we get 'is say so." Tom thought fast.

"Vis man's sick," he reported. "I've got ta git 'im ta ver boats: ve doctor said."

"Blimey, mate! The sorta sickness 'e's got must 'ave been caught out of a bottle. 'E's drunk: I kin smell 'im from 'ere."

"Naw, 'e's sick, I tell ya. Ve doctor said 'e was to 'ave a brandy, see: ta steady 'is nerves," persisted the unhappy Tom, not wanting to be involved in this argument, but also not wanting to lose face in front of his loved one.

"It's me dah," explained Sian. "E's sick: really like."

"E's drunk and 'e ain't going nowhere. And don't you give me any shit about the doctor, neither: 'e ain't got time to waste on the likes of 'im."

"Gi' us a chance, mate. 'e's me girl friend's dad," pleaded Tom, trying a new approach.

"Git back in line and wait yer turn like all the ouvers!" snapped a burly seaman from beside the steward. "You ain't going nowhere till the Captain says."

"Anyway, you can forget it," advised the steward. "They won't put 'im in a boat; not in that condition. There ain't enough places to go around now, and e's likely to die of cold before 'e even wakes up. You ain't got no chance, mate, when there's others more deservin' to be put off."

"Like them First Class toffs an' their snooty wives," raved Sian.

"I don't make the rules, love," the steward told her sadly, "I'm just 'ere to see 'em carried out." The seaman was not so understanding. He raised a balled fist and shouted.

"Look, you've bin told: now bugger off!" It was then Sian turned on Tom.

"Arn'cha gunna do something, like?" she demanded.

"Like what?" Tom asked, having to utilise all his strength to prevent Mick falling over.

"Yer a man, int yer? Push yer way through!" Sian commanded. Using the unwieldy Mick as a battering ram, Tom tried to force a passage between the steward and the seaman, but the seaman held his ground, raising his fist once more.

"Pack in shovin' or I'll do for ya," he warned. To his cost, Tom took no notice and continued to try and bulldoze Mick through a non existent gap. The crowd around them was unhelpful, shouting encouragement to the seaman.

"Smack ' im one, mate, 'e's jumpin' the queue."

"Don't let 'im get away with it."

"We were 'ere first: if anyone's goin' through, it should be us." The seaman delivered a backhand slap across Tom's face, as if he were returning a tennis ball across the net. The gnarled knuckles caught Tom on the nose and almost crushed it, which started it bleeding copiously. There came a sudden hiss from the crowd at the sight of violence: the simultaneous intake of a score of breaths, close by. Tom almost let Mick slip from his grasp at the shock of the blow, having to bend to hold the man as he slid towards the deck. It exposed his face entirely to the seaman who readied his arm to swing another punch. Tom closed his eyes and gritted his teeth. The strike never came.

"What's going on?" shouted a deep, resonant voice. Tom opened his eyes to see a man, all of six foot four tall, and dressed in a blue uniform, standing behind the seaman and looking over his shoulder. The Master at Arms had arrived, alerted by the disturbance.

"This man is trying to force 'is way up to the Boat Deck," reported the steward.

"I 'it 'im, cos it was the only way to stop 'im," the seaman explained, in an attempt to justify his actions. "This bloke 'ere is drunk - dead drunk - an' they're tryin' to git him to the boats before the ouvers."

"You'll have to wait your turn, sir," boomed the Master at Arms, supporting the crew, "and they'll not be taking any drunks in the boats. It is women and children first. You are wasting your time, sir." He sounded adamant.

"They'll not be takin' Third Class drunks," yelled Sian above the growing hubbub, "but I bet you 'alf them toffs are well plastered." A deep murmur of concordance swept through the crowd at her words and they pushed forward.

"Get back the lot of ya!" bawled the Master at Arms, and the crew closed ranks to keep them out, linking arms as they did so. "There will be no drunks in the lifeboats from any Class," the Master at Arms continued loudly with an explanation which would go over everybody's head, but still imparted a clear message. "Alcohol dehydrates the body, and they won't survive in the cold, so there's no point in taking them," and then he said to Tom, indicating Mick, "Get him out of here before I have my men throw him overboard. You'll have to wait your turn."

"Bastard! Pig!" Sian railed at him, and Tom tried to pull her away, burdened as he was by the immobile Liverpudlian.

"It's no good, gel, vey ain't gonna let 'im fru." Tom tried to console her. "C'mon, gel, let's git back to ve cabin. Maybe we kin sober 'im up, hey?"

"Do something. Yer can't let them leave me dah behind, like," she pleaded.

"What kin I do?" Tom demanded, eyeing the cordon of seamen. Bright blood was running down his chin and dripping onto his jacket. His hands were full and he could not wipe it away, even if he had owned a handkerchief to do it with.

"Yer bloody useless, yer are!" Sian screamed at him. "Just like all them other men!" The crowd around them quietened down, overawed by Sian's rage. "Get away from me; go back to yer bastard wife and all yer snotty kids. I'll luke after me dah on me own!" Unreasonably she tried to wrest her father from Tom's grasp but he held on grimly: thunderstruck.

"But I can't do anyfink, gel," he complained. "Vey won't let me."

"Clear off, leave 'im alone!" stormed the girl, renewing her efforts to drag her father clear.

"Hold up, gel! You know I love ya!" he shouted back, suddenly afraid of what she might say.

"Well, I don't love yer, yer pillock, an' I never did. Now clear off back to your bloody wife," she replied.

"But I'm comin' ta Chicago whiff ya," he reminded her lamely.

"No yer soddin' not," Sian retorted. Quite undismayed by fifty pairs of avidly listening ears, Sian laid it on the line for him. "I only wanted yer cos I didn't think me dah would hold down a job, like: I mean, luke at the state of 'im. I thought you could support us until I found a proper man. If they won't take me dah in the boats, an 'e's gunna die; whorra I need yer fur? I can find someone much better than you." Tom was flabbergasted.

"But Sian... gel... " he began.

"Clear off I tell yer, and stop callin' me bloody 'gel' like a silly arse. Go on, piddle off! Go on back to yer fat slut of a wife an' yer effin' squalid kids!" she screeched at him. The look of malevolent hate in her eyes could not be mistaken. Tom dropped the ponderous Mick and fled to the safety of the companionway.

The sight of an intruder in his stateroom enraged Lucas enormously, but he was not man enough to do much about it except resort to stinging invective.

"What the deuce do you think you are doing, Peacock?" he demanded while the surprise was still on him. The man had been unaware of his entrance, but turned around at the sound of his voice, looking very ashamed. David could not hold the gambler's eyes, flicking his gaze from floor to ceiling in an attempt to avoid his protagonist.

"You must know what I'm looking for," he explained quietly.

"You bloody gentry are all the same," Lucas accused. "You're born with a silver spoon in your mouth and you risk your life to get your money back when you've lost a few bob, fair and square."

"It was not fair and square," came back David stubbornly. "You cheated me!"

"Bosh! Stuff and nonsense! And that's something else I can't stand about people like you. You're so damned supercilious. Your forebears probably made a fortune out of slaving, or some such illegal trade, and you still think you're better than anyone else in the world. Well, you're not, Mr Sodding Peacock, and you've no right to look down on me! You made a bad error of judgement when you took me on, and because you lost you want to brand me as a cheat. Well, you carry on. You won't find your cheque because it is not in the bottom of the suitcase you are just about to vandalise. I suspected you might try something like this. I have it on my person and if you want it you'll have to come and get it... if you think you can." Lucas did not think David would try and he was right.

"Give it to me," said David, holding out his hand. "I want it back. You are wrong. My family did not make a fortune as you say: it had one two hundred years ago but lost it through bad management."

"It looks distinctly like it has lost a little more for the same reason," scoffed Lucas. "I don't know! You lose a few pennies and you will move heaven and earth to get it back. What is our gentry coming to?"

"It might only be a few pennies to you, but it is a great deal to me... all the money I have in the world, to support my wife and children." David was not pleading; merely putting the gambler straight. "It was dishonestly taken off me, whatever you might say, and I intend to have it back."

"Mr Peacock, you are in danger of breaking my heart. If I had known you would be here, I might have hired a few violin players to soothe your wounded breast." Lucas pushed his scorn to the limit. "You will be telling me next how your wife and children are doomed to end up in the workhouse."

"Not far off," David told him. "I don't know who you think I am, but I am certainly not from a wealthy family as you suggest. I am afraid you have preyed on the wrong man this time. I am in trade, sir, a lowly commercial traveller abroad on my employer's business. I cannot afford the sort of money you cheated me out of. I had thought we were playing a friendly game, amongst gentlemen, to pass away the time pleasantly. I had not expected to be comprehensively rooked of more than I could afford." Lucas was astounded. He had no idea David was in trade, and still did not quite believe it.

"Are you telling me the cheque is no good?" he demanded.

"No. It could be met, but it is not going to be, because you are going to give it me back. I have just told you it is all the money I have in the world and my wife and children are not going to suffer at your hands, Mr Meredith, whatever you may think." It sounded like a threat to Lucas, and he shifted uneasily on his feet. While he thought he had the upper hand he had not worried, but if this man spoke the truth, he was likely to do anything to protect his family. Perhaps the man was just a good liar!

"If you do not have much money, as you claim, how is it you are travelling First Class? I know what it costs and it doesn't seem likely that a man in your position, in trade, would be able to afford such luxury," Lucas refuted.

"My firm is paying the fare as a reward for my successes last year. I could not ordinarily afford to travel in this way. My wife and I were regarding it as a second honeymoon until you put paid to that idea with your skullduggery. I ought to wring your neck!" David had uttered the words with such conviction that Lucas was persuaded at last. He had really slipped up on his homework this time. If he had known David could not afford to lose, Lucas would never have entertained him at the table or set him up. Maybe he was slipping: perhaps it was time to give up? Then he remembered the condition of the ship and it did not seem to matter any more.

Lucas pulled the cheque from the inside pocket of the coat. He looked at the amount, and the payee, and smiled wryly. Then he tore the cheque into little pieces and walked towards David slowly. He made a great show of putting the shreds in the outstretched hand.

"There you are: there is your cheque. If you will take my advice, stay away from card schools if you cannot afford to lose: there are some funny people about in this world who are quick to take advantage." David looked down at the scraps of paper in his hand. The gambler's change of heart was totally unexpected. He had thought he would have to fight the man for the return of his money. Surprised as he was, he could think of nothing to say. Lucas had not expected thanks. He continued, "Now sir, if you don't mind, I should like you to vacate my stateroom: I do have pressing matters in hand." Lucas bent to pick up his clothes, which David had spilled onto the floor, and was stuffing them back into the case feverishly when David found his tongue.

"I can only thank you, Mr Meredith, for your consideration. Not for me, you understand, but for my wife and children." Lucas shook his head in disbelief.

"I can see now why you are in trade, though I can't understand, for the life of me, how you have made any success at it. You don't have to thank me, you fool! You were right: I cheated you, just as you said. Now, please, if you don't mind, I have urgent things to do, as I'm sure you have too."

However, David would just not go away. He stood his ground irritatingly.

"Why did you say I was risking my life to get my money back? It seems an odd remark," he mentioned. It was Lucas's turn to be surprised.

"Don't you know?" he asked.

"Know what?"

"The ship is about to sink. It has hit an iceberg: ripped open like a tin can by all accounts." Then he smiled again, ignominiously. "So you see, my gesture has not been so noble after all. I could hardly have shown your cheque around London, as I threatened, after the sea had washed off all the ink, could I?" Then Lucas laughed ironically.

"Are you sure?" David entreated.

"I have just come from speaking with the designer. I take it he should know. I don't suppose we've long to wait, by now. Shouldn't you be escorting your family to the boats?" David's face assumed an dismayed look as he accepted the gambler's intelligence as true.

"And you... are you coming?" David wanted to know, and suddenly Lucas knew the answer to that. What was it the designer had said, something about 'making his own judgement about how he had conducted his life before feeling he had any rights over the innocent'? He had hardly led an exemplary life, conniving and cheating his way through it, for more years than he cared to remember, and was not of much account in the final analysis. What right had he to push his case when this innocent stood before him; a patsy who had thanked him for returning ill gotten gains? Better this young man took his place in the lifeboat with his wife and children, giving them the chance to live on in the comfort of his indispensable support.

"I think not," he announced, "though I am touched by your concern for my welfare after I have admitted cheating you."

"If you are right and the ship is going to sink directly, come with me and at least try and save yourself, for God's sake. It is not the time for recriminations," David insisted, but Lucas shook his head.

"After my interview, with the Captain, today, concerning my treatment of you, I suspect I shall be the last man they will put in the boats, of which there are not enough to go round, or so the designer says. I am persona non grata now, you see. Save yourself, and your family, and do not worry on my account. Whether I survive or not will be my last great gamble in life."

"Mr Meredith, come on," urged David, too humane to see anyone perish needlessly. "I am sure everyone will get a fair crack of the whip in these unusual circumstances. I think that you are wrong."

"No, I think not," dissented the gambler. "I still have a few pages of my book to finish and can only hope I have time enough left to do so." He picked up the novel from the chair and smiled benignly. "Rider Haggard is such a good author, don't you think, and I'd like to see how the story comes out in the end."

Captain Arthur Rostron, of the Cunard Line's *Carpathia* was sound asleep when the news of the *Titanic's* predicament was brought to him. At first, he did not believe his ears.

"Good God! The *Titanic*... sinking... are you sure?" he asked to have the fact that this was not a bad dream, swiftly verified.

"Yes sir, according to the distress signal they are putting out," he was told by the officer who had awakened him.

"Have they said what's wrong?"

"Yessir, they've hit an iceberg and are badly holed." Captain Rostron was up in a flash and pulling on his uniform.

"Have they given their position?" He continued to fire questions at the officer as he dressed hurriedly.

"Yessir."

"Well, man?"

"They are at Lat 41... "

"No, man... I meant, have you worked it out?" complained Rostron. "How far are they away from our present position?"

"About fifty-eight miles, sir: nor-nor-west."

"Good God! As far as that?"

"I'm afraid so, sir. What shall I tell them? They're sending all the time."

"Tell them... " Rostron thought for a moment. "Tell them we are coming at full speed. Pray God we will be there in time... but don't tell them that last bit!"

Harold Bride delivered the intelligence to the bridge and the Captain was already on his way to the Marconi Room before he had managed to get it all out. Jack Phillips was crouched over his set, fingers flying on the morse key; the radio shack buzzing to the sound of the angry, urgent code.

"You have raised a ship then?" asked the Captain anxiously.

"Yessir. The *Carpathia*. I am calling her now." The senior operator's left hand continued to oscillate furiously while his right hand was poised, pen clutched between nervous fingers, to write down what he received.

"What are they saying?" demanded the Captain. Phillips' hand paused, hovering above the key as he listened and then began to write.

"They say they have turned the ship around and are coming at full speed."

"How long will they be? How far are they away?" The Captain spouted out his questions but had to wait for an answer, as Phillips began transmitting again.

"She says she will be here in about three and a half hours," the operator reported pessimistically, and the Captain's heart sank; the flame of hope extinguished in a flood of renewed distress. The receiver continued to chatter. "They say they will make all possible speed and ask us to hold on, as best we can, until they arrive."

The Captain turned away so the disappointment, on his features, was hidden from the two men. If Andrews was right, the ship did not have that long to live. Just how long could he keep the ship afloat? What could he do, that had not already been done, to slow down the rate of water-seepage? While he grappled with the problem, another promising thought occurred to him.

"Ask her where she is," he ordered Phillips, and waited patiently for the reply.

"To the south east, sir, outward bound from New York." The little spark of optimism, still alive in the Captain's breast, was breathed back into life once more. The *Carpathia* was in the right direction, and only forty-eight miles from the *Titanic's* true position. She could be here in three hours or maybe less, depending on what speed she could make, although the Captain knew she could not match the awesome power of his own engines. An outside chance still existed that help could arrive on time, and he threw himself back into his role with enthusiasm - while there is probability, there is always hope.

"What about this other ship: the one you said was close?" he interrogated impatiently.

"I don't know, sir, I haven't been able to raise her yet," admitted Phillips.

"Her bloody operator must be asleep or drunk. We should be almost blowing her out of the water with the strength of our calls. Keep trying... oh... and call the *Carpathia* again, and tell her to come as fast as she can for pity's sake. Tell her we have not got enough lifeboats aboard to get everyone off. We need her here, soon, if more than half our complement of passengers and crew are to survive."

Back on the bridge, the Captain called over the Sixth Officer.

"You can start sending off those distress-rockets now. Fire one every fifteen minutes. Keep firing them until I tell you to stop."

"Yes, sir. Does this mean help is on the way?" The boy was irrepressible!

"Yes, and we can only pray it will be here in time." The Captain stared out of the bridge window when the officer had gone, into the north, hoping he might yet spot the lights of the phantom ship, somewhere out there in the darkness but there was no sign. Then, reluctantly, he decided to send a message to the officers on the Boat Deck, telling them to load up the women and children. The time had come to get them off the ship.

Lorna, with Nanny's assistance, shepherded the gaggle of children, and her ineffectual husband, up the Grand Staircase, to the Boat Deck, on top of the superstructure. Where one would expect chaos, there was only order. The orchestra played soothing melodies from a point close by, which drifted over the assembled passengers and out into the cold night air. The crowd stood patiently in the centre of the deck, already incorporating a forward slant, and watched the preparations, as the lifeboats were made ready to be launched, hanging out over the side of the ship in their arched davits. Everyone wore a canvas life preserver, and the atmosphere was as calm as that of a garden party. Little knots of people stood about, chatting, as if they were waiting to be presented to the guest of honour.

It was not a scene to reinstate any of Lorna's earlier fears; surely there could be no danger here. It must be as the Steward had said to her husband: over zealous precautions by a conscientious Captain, mindful of his passengers' well-being. She even paused to exchange a word with the American couple who shared their dining table.

"Isn't it exciting?" breezed the woman. "We've never experienced an emergency before." She looked comical in her bulky jacket, tied round her body with long strings; but then Lorna realised she must appear quite ridiculous herself.

"Well, not exactly exciting," she disavowed. "More of a nuisance, really. I would much rather be tucked up in bed."

"You don't think the ship will sink, then?" inquired the man.

"Good Lord, no. My husband assures me it is the safest ship afloat, and he should know: he is a scientist. Look at him, he is quite calm! I shouldn't think there is anything to worry about." The American gentleman looked relieved: it was apparent he did not share his wife's liking for this sort of thrill.

Jonathan was far from calm inside, where it mattered. His mind had switched off from the trauma he knew was to come, and abject fear bubbled around inside him. In his safe academic sphere, he had never contemplated such a tragedy would impinge on his life - and he was convinced by what he had seen of its workings, and construction, that the *Titanic* would go down like a stone at any minute - the only previous danger he had encountered being when an experiment he was conducting had gone dangerously wrong. Plucked from his safe world, where life was so monotonously predictable, he could not imagine how any of them could be saved from the death throes of this shattered, steel monstrosity. He had never looked death in the face before, or even contemplated it, and the prospect short-circuited contradictory brain cells, leaving him in a cataleptic state, no longer able to face up to the reality of the situation. This cathartic condition robbed him of the power of reason and he had to be led about, and directed, like a autistic child; much more an island, in himself, than he had ever been before.

"Lorna, Lorna... " The urgent cries attracted Lorna's attention and she searched the crowd, to find Molly rushing towards her.

"Oh, you've bought the children with you. How good of you to think like that!" Molly greeted.

"Well, when no one came for them, I thought I better had. Nanny had them ready, of course, so we came up here together." Her remark was not one of censure, but Molly apparently took it so.

"But David was coming for the children," Molly explained. "He told me to come up here, directly, while he fetched them." Then an expression of horror invaded her face. "You mean he never arrived! Have you seen him? Did you see him anywhere; on the way, perhaps?"

"No, I'm afraid not," Lorna said forlornly. "I had my hands full with the children, of course, but saw neither hide nor hair of him. He never came to the stateroom while we were there."

"What could have happened to him?" wailed Molly and the implications of the thought almost destroyed her previous composure. "Do you think he might be lying injured somewhere? I think I had better go and look for him."

"You will do no such thing!" Lorna heard herself say. "You must stay here with your children and look after them. I am sure no harm has come to... your husband. Perhaps, he has lost his way or been delayed. Molly, dear, your children need you here. I am sure he will come at any moment."

"Yes, I am sure you are right," Molly agreed, only partially comforted. "I was being a bit silly..." Then she knew instinctively where David had gone. It explained his stifling of the situation: the recent lack of information from him. In his anger and remorse, Molly perceived, he had gone to face the man who cheated him, yet again, in an attempt to recover his losses. Molly was suddenly very afraid, and she pictured him lying in a cabin, not unlike their own, badly injured or worse: battered by the monster, Meredith, she conjured up in her imagination. She had to go and find him, and opened her mouth to explain the situation to Lorna when she was interrupted. Her words were never uttered.

"Come on, ladies, it is time to board the boats." The First Officer had arrived at their side; anxiously trying to marshall uncooperative passengers.

"Is it really necessary?" challenged Lorna.

"Captain's orders, ma'am: you are to get in the boats," the First Officer confirmed. "Are these your children?... yes... well, we must get them away to safety... now. Come on ladies, please," he added imperatively. No one had shown any inclination to board the lifeboats and the lack of attention to his orders was beginning to frustrate him: as First Officer, he was not amused by recalcitrance of any sort.

"But my husband is not here," protested Molly. "I cannot get in a boat: I must go and find him!"

"No, Molly," advised Lorna. "He will be alright. You must think of the children now. Come on... come along with Nanny and me: I am sure your David will soon turn up quite unharmed."

"Yes, why don't you do what the lady says," encouraged the First Officer, and Molly's conviction wavered, allowing Lorna to gather up her extended family and herd them towards the Boat Deck rail, much to the officer's satisfaction. However, his triumph would be short lived.

"I am sorry, it's women and children only," he had to tell Lorna as she pushed the comatose Jonathan to the fore. It was Lorna's turn to protest.

"But, he is my husband! I cannot go without him!" she insisted and clung to Jonathan's hand desperately; determined not to be separated from him.

"I'm sorry, ma'am... Captain's orders... women and children first."

"Then I shall not go," Lorna told him stubbornly. "I do not intend to leave him behind, and nor will my children." She began to pull her daughters back from the lifeboat, still yawningly empty in front of them.

"Madam, please... Get into the boat," ordered the First Officer, rapidly beginning to lose his patience.

"I will not... not without my, husband," Lorna objected.

"I think we can make an exception," said a voice from beside them. The Chairman had heard the commotion and come over to investigate. He had witnessed the contretemps.

"No sir," argued the First Officer. "The Captain was most specific: it is women and children first." The Chairman smiled at Lorna knowingly, giving her the distinct impression everything would be alright.

"Look at the man," he said to the officer in an aside. "You can see he is in a state of shock. Put him in the boat with his wife and children."

"I won't go without him," repeated Lorna pedantically, metaphorically stamping her foot.

"No sir," reiterated the First Officer, "the Captain said... "

"The devil take the Captain!" roared the Chairman, not happy to be dismissed. "I am the Chairman of this Line, and I say you will put him in the boat." The First Officer looked from the Chairman to Jonathan and back, uncertainly. Then he shrugged and turned to the seamen beside him.

"Put them in the boat," he capitulated.

"But my husband is not here," submitted Molly. "Can you hold the lifeboat while I go and look for him?" The Chairman beamed his most charming smile.

"That is not possible, madam: time is tight. But do not worry, dear lady, there is room enough for everyone. We shall have your husband loaded into another boat as soon as all you women and children are away. You have my word," he assured her, and placated, Molly gave up the one-sided struggle.

Strong hands helped them into Starboard No 7, which would be the first lifeboat away. It would leave with twenty-eight people on board, when its capacity was sixty-five, because no one else could be persuaded to enter it. Indifference would work against the crew's efforts to save the passengers, as they showed no urgency to save themselves - most of them still believing the fiction of the *Titanic's* invulnerability, and that she would never founder. As the boat was lowered towards the dark sea, eighty feet below, the strained, white faces of the occupants looked up dubiously; still not sure they were doing the right thing by leaving, until they became ghostlike in the gloom. Only Nanny appeared to be taking the whole thing seriously, sitting in the stern with her arms folded across the cork bolster which swelled out her already ample chest.

David Peacock arrived at the Second Class cabin where his children were berthed, to find the door wide open and the children gone. He had lost all track of time while he delayed in Meredith's cabin, and was rather surprised to find the stateroom empty. He wandered in and found it had been left as if the children, and Nanny, had simply vanished. Toys littered the floor where they had obviously been playing earlier: John's bright lead soldiers and Rebecca's expensive French doll.

Perplexed, he wandered about the cabin making further checks. Their clothes were still in the chest of drawers, and their beds rumpled as if they have been used. Then he remembered it was late, and that they had probably been roused from sleep: but where would they have gone without him? Just then, he had the presence of mind to look up to the top of the wardrobe and noticed the life-jackets had vanished as well. Of course, Nanny would have taken them up to the Boat Deck, and they had probably been reunited with Molly by now. He visibly relaxed. With old Nanny in charge, they were in the best hands imaginable. Feeling rather redundant, he set off in search of his family.

He had not come down to the children's cabin that frequently, leaving their welfare to Molly, as was normal at the time, and was disorientated by the unfamiliarity of the Second Class accommodation's warren of gangways and passages. As a consequence, he soon lost his way. He rounded a corner, in search of the stair-well, and came upon a firmly-locked, expandable steel gate across the passageway. It had been padlocked from the side he was on - top and bottom - and was a formidable barrier, as he was just about to find out. As he stood there, trying to recover his bearings, a mob of frantic people howled down the gangway towards him, on the other side of the gate, and seemed to throw themselves against it in anxiety, although it was the press of the crowd behind which gave this impression. The gate held under the impact and the charge was stemmed.

They stood there for a long, long second, David and the forerunners, staring at each other in amazement, each of them confused by the sudden encounter: David with the mob, and the mob with the gate. A tall, dark haired young man was conspicuous in the van, and it was he who recovered his composure first. He stretched out an arm, through the latticed steel, and snatched at David's lapel; a move David only just managed to avoid. He wished for no contact with the hoi polloi, and these people, by their dress, were obviously steerage passengers.

"'Elp us, guv: please," pleaded the young man. "We're tryin' ta git ta ve Boat Dick!" David recoiled from the hand which still groped for him. The man appeared to have been involved in some sort of fracas, as there was carapaces of dried blood on his upper lip and chin, and dark blobs, of the same substance, stained the front of his coat. The eyes which were fixed on David were terrible: suffused with great anger and immeasurable hurt, as if he had been deeply wounded by life.

"What can I do?" David asked uncertainly.

"Find somefink ta 'elp us break darn vis gate," suggested the young man.

"Exactly what did you have in mind?" David wanted to know, trying to maintain his dignified front.

"I dunno," snapped the voluble young man. "A crow-bar; anyfink; somefink like vat." David looked down at his clothes.

"I do not usually carry anything like that in my evening suit," he informed the East Ender. The young man's face clouded with hatred at the gibe.

"Doan piss abaut, mate," he berated David. "If we can't git fru vis effing gate, we're all gunna draan," and he rattled the barrier in an attempt to emphasise his point. The seriousness of their predicament was brought home to David in no uncertain terms. He noticed several women in the crowd, and his gentlemanly instincts told him he must do something to help them.

He stepped forward and examined the padlocks. They were heavy and solid looking, and without the keys, or some heavy instrument, there would be no chance of getting them off. Whoever had closed this barrier, did not want these people to get past.

"Hang on," he said, directing his words to the young man. "I'll see if I can find someone with a key."

"Vat's naw bleedin' good!" complained the spokesman. "Vey wanta keep us aut, see, so vey ain't likely ta give ya no keys, are vey? If ya gonna 'elp us, mate, you'll 'ave to find a crowbar or a pieca metul from somewhere."

David looked around himself desperately: it was alright to say that, but where would he find what the young man was asking for.

"Hang on, I will see what I can do," he muttered, and fled around the corner. Away from the intensity of the crowd, his enthusiasm for their plight began to wane. Everyone he spoke to was convinced the ship was about to sink, and he had not found his family yet. He did not know where they were or what had happened to them. Yet, he was loath to run off on his own selfish mission and leave those unfortunates to a terrible fate. He dithered on the edge of indecision. Should he do what they wanted, or abandon them to their destiny; saving himself in the process? His conscience made the judgement for him, and he set off to see what he could find. It would be a long, drawn-out process.

Most of the staterooms about him had been abandoned in haste, and the doors had been left wide open. He rushed in and out of the cabins searching for something - anything - which might help the steerage passengers. What he sought was obviously not a common item to carry on a sea voyage. He found an iron bound chest in one of the staterooms, with iron ribs which looked hefty enough to suit their purpose, but after a great deal of straining, with his considerable strength, was unable to dislodge them from their seating. He gave up and moved on. It was in the umpteenth cabin he visited that he finally found the only thing which might fit the bill. It was a sturdy metal frame, the like of which he had not seen before, crudely constructed for some obscure purpose. It was about three foot tall, with four distinct legs, and two handles which stuck out backwards from the structure, with just about enough room for a human body to fit in between them. However, he had no time to assess what its true purpose might be, and snatched it up, to carry it off to the barrier in the passageway.

When he arrived, he perceived he had another problem. Not wanting to delay here longer than necessary, for purely selfish reasons, he found there was no way to pass the cumbersome frame through to the young man beyond the gate.

"Yule 'ave ta break orf ve padlocks from vat side," counselled the man. David sighed in discontent: he did not want to be here doing this. He had hoped to find something and hand it over to let them do the job: he was not a man to welcome manual labour. Nevertheless, he lifted up the frame and lodged two of the legs into the skeleton of the gate, behind the top padlock. He took up the strain and pulled with all his might, but to no avail: the stubborn metal, or its fixings, would not budge.

"Git ya feet up an va wall," advised the young man, avidly watching every move. "It'll gi' ya more leverage," and David followed his instructions. He strained and he heaved, employing one leg against the wall, and then both, until his body was off the ground. He pulled and he grappled, until dark veins of effort stood out on his forehead, and the muscles of his chest and neck were rigidly defined. Then there came an audible crack, and the frame disintegrated in his hands. He fell back into the passage heavily, bruising his back in the process. The frame fell an top of him and stabbed him in the groin.

As he lay there, smarting from the pain, he knew he had endured enough on these people's behalf. He picked himself up slowly.

"Ya awhite, mate?" called out the young man, obviously concerned. David looked down and saw his makeshift tool had broken into two pieces; the metal shiny in places, at the breaks, but substantially ingrained with dull flaws. He did no more than pick up the two manageable halves and pass them through the gate to the young man.

"You will have to break it down yourself," he wheezed through his damaged chest. "I cannot stay any longer: I've got to find my family, you understand?" He could not avoid the clutching hand this time, as it was painful to move suddenly, and it grabbed hold of his jacket and held him... for a few moments. David's being filled with apprehension; he had done what he could, what did they want of him now?

"Fanks, guv: yore a gent," said the young man earnestly in genuine appreciation; not a comment of rancour. The hand released him.

"I'm sorry," muttered David in remorse, "but I must go... my family... they need me."

"Good luck, guv: I 'ope va Good Lord looks arter ya," the young man told him with sincerity, and David fled; back the way he had come.

He found the staircase at the second attempt, and ran up it towards the Boat Deck at full speed, ignoring the pain in his chest which caused him agony when he breathed; suggesting broken ribs. The determination to see Molly and the children safe, drove him on. He emerged at the top; into a sea of humanity. The Boat Deck was packed, and he could see no sign of his wife in the milling crowd. He ran forward and began to search each female face desperately. He had missed the launching of Starboard No 7 lifeboat by two minutes.

The Chairman was in his element: using his authority and influence to dictate the fate of the people around him, as was his special talent. He enjoyed the electric buzz of having the power of life and death in his hands, which smacked of perverted sexuality - although he would never recognise it as such, merely enjoying its stimulating impact.

He searched through the crowd for his cronies and acquaintances - as well as prestigious passengers he did not want suing the Line - and led them to the safety of the boats, and emancipation from the *Titanic's* likely fate. It was an unequivocal case of unprincipled favouritism, but he was not unduly concerned about that, as long as he got his way. The First Officer was putty in his hands, and in awe of his lofty position, but the Second Officer was not as pliable, objecting volubly to the Chairman's interference in his lifesaving operations. The Second Officer was following his Captain's orders to the letter. As a consequence, most of the favoured escapees were being channelled out through the boats on the starboard side. There was a more ominous reason, now, for the lifeboats going away undermanned: the Chairman was ordering them off half-filled to protect his interests: he could not afford to have the craft swamped, and see his carefully conceived work demolished. He had long since realised the super-rich passengers would not sue for damages, over an unavoidable accident, if they came through the ordeal safely; although their families might do so if they perished. Trying as hard as he could to save his Company's neck, much of the Chairman's efforts were being negated by the Second Officer, who was refusing all, but the women and children, access to the port-side boats. The Second Officer would maintain his stand until the bitter end. Many a privileged, and furious gentleman would be turned away by this stickler for the rules of the sea.

Things were just not going right for poor Tom, and he watched David scamper away from the gate with conflicting emotions, which only added to the miasma he had already experienced during the day. The pain from the smack in the nose that he had received from the seaman had long since receded - although he still had difficulty breathing through the dried encrustations clogging his nostrils - but the humiliation lingered on. Then there was his unbelievable rejection, at the hands of Sian - when he had pledged his all to her - to be contended with; plus the outrage and indignity of being taken for a fool, and used for convenience purposes by a conniving woman. Piled on top of this was the considerable remorse he suffered for breaking faith with Amy, at the first sniff of a willing quim, after all these years, when she had been his comfort and joy for so long. Throwing the anxiety he felt for her safety, and that of the kids, into the melting pot, had concocted a powerful brew: a heady stew of over-wound muscle and sinew, and seething rage, hanging fire on a very short fuse. It was only the unexpected help he had elicited from the gentleman, on the other side of the gate, which had stayed the match to set him off in a violent explosion of temper, coloured by hatred, fury and self disgust.

After his brutal dismissal by the girl, he had dived down into the bowels of the ship, to escape further embarrassment, knowing there was no way forward up on deck; and desperate to get to the bow, where he had left Amy in bed. All his ardent sensations of love for her had returned in the moment of rejection by Sian, and he wondered how he could have been so easily deceived, and why he had followed his adulterous appetites to the very edge of a precipice.

Down below, he had found his way blocked at every turn. The throughways, of the upper decks - in First and Second Class - were locked off by the barred gates, and deeper down, forward progress was prevented by the rising waters, flooding into the ship. Deeply frustrated by failure, he had eventually run into a group of steerage passengers - running around and seeking escape, like a flock of headless chickens - and assumed command, deciding a small force was better than single effort; if he could get them all working together for the common good. He had managed to succeed. Now as he stood there, with the strangely-shaped pieces of metal in his hands, he was eternally grateful to the man - now hastily, and understandably, departed for giving them the means, and the chance to save themselves from the turbid flood which threatened to engulf them from below.

Tom took stock of their position. The locking side of the security gate, on which the gentleman had worked, was too firmly fixed to the wall, by the look of it, to succumb to easy demolition. The other side, where the gate was anchored, appeared to be a much better prospect. The brackets, which held the gate upright, were bolted into the wood panelling of the corridor, and did not exhibit insurmountable difficulties.

"C'mon mates," he urged his team of willing helpers. "Let's git va gates orf from vis side." He handed out the weird iron bars, and superintended the efforts of the men; giving out with helpful comments, as he saw the need. "Stick va bars in vere, behind va uprights, see... no, put vat piece rand vere... now 'eave, willya... c'mon, mates, put ya bicks inta it."

Several men hung on each bar, top and bottom, until with a rending crack of splitting wood, the upper bracket gave up the uneven struggle, and the gate sagged.

"All tagivver naa," encouraged Tom. "Jess one more good 'eave, lads." The wood capitulated and they were through: the barrier casually tossed aside in the process. They charged on down the passageways, in the body of the ship, looking for a way out: spilling out onto the Boat Deck, a few minutes later, by way of the Second Class Staircase, and lunging on towards the port-side boats. Tom was more concerned about peeling off to find Amy, but was carried along with the tide, at the head of his agitated troops. They might have swamped the nearest boat - presently being loaded with passengers - had not an officer - supremely cool under pressure - stepped out in front of them and raised his hands.

"Get back!" he commanded, "it's women and children first." The rampaging mob of steerage passengers took no heed of his words, or actions, and pressed forwards: one of the men, in the van, still clutching an iron bar, from the frame, and preparing to swat the officer with it.

An ugly looking revolver appeared suddenly in the Second Officer's hand, and the deafening reports from the two warning shots, he fired over the mob's head, brought everything on the Boat Deck to a abrupt stop: even the orchestra, which ground to a ragged halt.

"Get back... or I fire!" shouted the officer, with another warning. "It's women and children first, I tell you." The snubby muzzle of the weapon fell to point directly at Tom, and he stood where he had stopped, at the shock of the gunfire: dead still. His surrounding henchmen cringed away, leaving him to the fore, exposed, as if he were the only culprit. Every eye on the Boat Deck turned on him, accusingly. "Now get back," threatened the Second Officer, waving him away with the pistol. "You will get your turn when the women and children are safely away."

Tom pivoted, bitterly ashamed, and slunk away in search of his family.

The lifeboats went away one by one, as the bow settled deeper and deeper into the water. The *Titanic* was beginning to show a definite list to port by now, as the water, restricted by the compartmentalised fabric of the ship, filled up the hull unevenly: the deck canting to an uncomfortable degree. The first boat to go, No 6, on the port-side, was lowered into the sea at twelve fifty-five, with only twenty-eight people on board. The Chairman flitted from one side of the Boat Deck to the other, encouraging his chosen few to enter, and urging the officers to get them away at once. He would suffer several disappointments! Passengers still did not comprehend the ship was doomed to sink and the well bred, and mannered, amongst them, stood back to see what would transpire from this orderly confusion. The Fifth Officer, loading starboard No. 5, objected vehemently to the Chairman interfering with his command, but the Chairman won in the end by pulling rank, and the boat went away with forty on board; twenty-four short of its actual capacity.

Starboard No. 3 was lowered with only thirty-two passengers in the seats, and the prime example of the Chairman's machinations, starboard No. 1 - with space for forty - was launched with only twelve in place. It was understandable as the English Lord and his designer wife were the VIP's aboard, with seven of the crew to make sure they came to no harm. They would, as personal friends of the Chairman, be the only passengers to be called at the British Board of Trade Inquiry, and would back him to the hilt; confirming everything the Chairman told them about the disaster, at the time and subsequently, as if they had seen it with their own eyes.

Port-side No. 8 was lowered containing only thirty-nine people. The Second Officer had loaded it with all the available women and children he could find, but would not break the rigid order of, 'women and children first', he had received from the Captain, so directed it away as it was. Ida Strauss could have been aboard, along with the Countess of Rothes, but when her husband, Isador, was refused entry by the Second Officer, she turned away, saying to him lovingly, "We have been living together for so many years: where you go, I go!" The magnificent couple calmly sat down in two deck chairs to watch and wait for another opportunity; which would never come. The formidable Countess of Rothes, however, took to her new situation like a duck to water. With only one seaman in the boat, she took the tiller and eventually assumed command: usurping the rights of her fellow-sufferers, as only a British aristocrat can do. The King's subjects, with her, accepted her lien, out of innate familiarity with a traditional system, whether she was right or wrong, and the

Americans, without a nobility of their own, blatantly encouraged her to govern their destiny, and their fate.

The fact that the Chairman's policy of flagrant discrimination worked, would be born out by the survival statistics. Of the twenty-nine children in the First and Second Class, twenty-eight would survive the disaster. Only one, three year old Lorraine Allison of Montreal - who clung to the skirts of a mother who would not leave a husband behind - would be unaccounted for. Fifty-three out of the seventy-six children in the Steerage would perish with the ship: their lives wantonly cut off by prejudice, and the hypothermic cold of the sea. It was not a pleasant result for anyone to have on their conscience!

As time went by, little, niggling voices, inside the Chairman's head, began to suborn his good intentions.

"Why should you die?" they asked, and "Surely, of all the people on board, you have the power, the authority and the right to save yourself and live?" Suddenly he knew he had never intended to go down with the ship, despite what he had told the Captain. Who on the Board of Directors could replace him at the helm of the Company, or stand up to the storm which was about to break around their ears at the loss of the *Titanic*? He could think of no one: no person he could safely entrust with the continuance of the White Star Line. From this moment on, he looked for an opportunity to get himself away to the relative safety of the lifeboats he was so diligently helping to load.

The Captain, forward on the bridge, was also having second thoughts about his role in the disaster, as bad reports on the *Titanic's* condition continued to flood in: it was bad news from every quarter. That he would be blamed for not taking better care of his ship, he had no doubts. That there were insufficient lifeboats, to carry off all the passengers and crew, would be laid at someone else's door; and he hoped it would be the Chairman's.

He came, slowly, to the notion, if he was to be blamed, it might as well be for the true facts rather than the Chairman's inventions. No help had arrived and he already knew the *Titanic* would not live long enough for the *Carpathia,* rushing towards them at full speed, to be of any great assistance, other than to pick up the lifeboats, and any other survivors fortunate enough to defeat the most wicked of elements.

Yet, it still stuck in his craw, that the Chairman might blacken his character with vile calumny: like reports of cowardice and necessary replacement, when the chips were down. It was not the fitting reward he sought, after so many years of faithful service, to the White Star Line, to have his memory so abused. He tried desperately hard to think of a way to circumvent the Chairman's deception, and put the matter right for the sake of history. It was entirely his own fault the ship had sailed, from Belfast, with a fire on board - he should have put his foot down firmly at the time, whatever the personal cost - and he was prepared to accept the blame for that, because it was a culpability the discerning public would accept: that he acted on orders from a superior. That his memory would be pilloried, for the sake of the Chairman's deviousness, was something he could not, and the very idea of it rankled deep within him.

If he could have the Chairman removed from his position of privilege, and hypothetically gagged by isolation, then it might be possible to limit the damage to his reputation, and his memory as a good Captain, despite this one error of judgement. Yet, how was it to be done? He could hardly have the Chairman removed from the Boat Deck, kicking and screaming, in full view of the passengers - God knows what the man would say during the process! Then there was the matter of loyalty to be considered. The Master at Arms' allegiance had already been seduced by promises of advancement and survival if the Chairman was to believed - and the only officers he had left on the bridge were the Third and the Sixth. Could he entrust such a task to them; a situation requiring them to lay constraining hands on the Chief Executive of the Line at a Captain's behest? Would they even consider following his orders? The Captain was not at all sure they would: they were so young and vital, and the Lord only knew what they had been offered, by the Chairman, during his absences in the radio shack. Before he made any move, he would have to give the matter careful, and further, consideration. The greatest satisfaction, he had, was in knowing the Chairman would die with him, and would not live to continue with his obnoxious variety of dishonesty.

It was inevitable, as they were on the same errand - finding missing families - Tom Pirbright and David Peacock should meet up again, and recognise each other.

"So you got through, then... through the gate," David greeted, when they came face to face at the rear of the Boat Deck.

"Yas," confirmed Tom, and then added, when he had identified his saviour, "Fanks fir va 'elp, guv."

"My pleasure... It was the least I could do in the circumstances," returned David pleasantly, as if he was addressing a customer, grateful over the receipt of a favour. A short uncomfortable silence followed. It was Tom who broke the ice.

"Did ya find ya family, guv?"

"No," replied David mournfully. "I can only assume they have been taken off the ship already, although I can find no one to confirm such a supposition."

"Naw, me niever: I int fand mine yit," Tom stated at cross purposes, not really listening keenly as his eyes continued to search the crowd, explaining as he did so. "I doan know where me missus kin be. We were in va steerage, see Guv, an' vey seem ta want ta keep likes of us orf vis dick." David appeared concerned at the thought.

"Surely not?" he postulated.

"Look at me nose, guv: it's what one of vem did ta me, when I tried ta git up ere earlier." Tom pointed to the damaged area with an index finger. "Where is your cabin?" asked David, wishing to change the subject: not keen to hear what this poor man was saying.

"Up va front: in va bows," reported Tom. David looked in that stricken direction and frowned.

"Oh dear!" he exclaimed. "Perhaps it is just they have not made it up to this deck yet."

"Naw, not whiff vem bleedin' locked gates in va road," complained Tom. David was loath to admit, to himself, such discrimination could be practised in these circumstances even after seeing the evidence with his own eyes.

"They might be trapped somewhere below and... " he began, but paused when an idea hit him. "Look, old chap... I mean... well, my family are probably safe while yours might be in danger. I have nothing to do except wait, so, if you like, I will come along with you; to help you look below. I do not know your good lady of course, but two heads are better than one... eh... and you might need some help, if you encounter more of those gates along the way." David Peacock had found his social conscience, and the task would occupy a troubled mind: what if his own family were trapped and had never made it to the Boat Deck?

"Would ya, guv?" exclaimed Tom in complete surprise, and gratitude. "I might need some 'elp at vat!"

"Come on: let us get started before it is too late," suggested David, already regretting voicing his idea. The pain in his broken ribs was such he did not fancy heavy exertion of any sort. Tom turned away, saying, "'Ang on a mo, guv."

"Where are you going?" demanded David in consternation, wanting to get on with the search now he was committed by his garrulous mouth. Tom turned back with a wry grin on his sharp features.

"I'm jist poppin' orf to see me mates, ta git vem funny iron bars ya fand," he explained. "Wait 'ere, guv: I'll be right bick,"

And so was formed a most unlikely partnership, which would endure until the end of the ship's life: an event not so far away.

The maiden voyage of the 'Greatest Ship Afloat' was nearing its end. The water had reached the name, *Titanic,* on the bow, and now she was beginning to list to starboard as the sea found a way into compartments which had stayed dry before, on the other side of the ship. The entire bow section was waterlogged and strove to sink under the weight of the thousands of tons of saline fluid inside her, while the stern section tried to resist the unnatural motion and float as normal; placing enormous strain on the fabric of the ship at a point where the third funnel rose out of the super-structure, just abaft mid-ship. As Thomas Andrews had dolefully forecast, the Atlantic Ocean poured inexorably into each virginal, watertight compartment as soon as the previous one was filled, and it would not be long before the tremendous load the *Titanic* was taking in overpowered the buoyancy of the air left inside her.

Naturally, as the deck canted more steeply, some urgency was transmitted to the Boat Deck by the unfamiliar posture of the liner. The remaining boats were sent away with more potential survivors than previously. Port-side No. 12 was lowered with forty women and children on board, and No. 14 with as many as sixty. The Fifth Officer had to contend with the first sign of panic from the previously disdainful First and Second Class passengers, and had to fire his pistol in the air to prevent the boat being swamped. Port-side No. 16

contained fifty people and Starboard No. 13, sixty-four: a full load. A terrible accident, which would have added to the cost in human life, was narrowly avoided when starboard No. 15 was almost lowered on top of No. 13, which had not yet cleared the ship's side. Only sterling work, by the seamen, aboard for the passengers' protection, got it clear by the narrowest of margins.

Up in the Marconi Room, Jack Phillips was still sending out bulletins to the fleet of ships in radio range. At one thirty-five, he reported faithfully, "We are sinking fast. Women and children in the boats. Cannot last much longer." It was a plea many would hear but none could do anything about.

Most of the forward boats were away by now, and the waiting passengers moved unconsciously towards the stern as it seemed to be the best bet for survival. The four collapsible boats were, at last, being readied for launching: they would be the last chance for passengers to get away and competition for places would be fierce.

The Captain had come to a momentous decision, although it was not one for which he greatly cared. If he could not trust in the loyalty of his officers, to apprehend the Chairman for him, he must resort to guile and deception, as the Chairman himself employed, to silence him. Once he had the man on the bridge, the Captain could keep him here, incommunicado, by any means, fair or foul, even if it meant physical involvement in the process. The Captain was not a small man, and had the burly Quartermaster, who was still at his post, to call upon if needed: knowing the seaman, at least, had not been 'got at' by the Chairman, and was likely to follow orders unquestioningly. The technicalities, of how it would be done, did not matter for the moment: the means would be found as the situation developed.

The Captain knew he had to find a way to supplant the Chairman's current interest, and bring him here post-haste and unsuspecting. He believed he had found the right formula.

"Third," he called out, and the officer hurried over. "Find the Chairman, out on the Boat Deck, will you? Give him my compliments and ask him to come to the bridge at once. Tell him... tell him the Marconi Room has located a steamer close at hand, and I need to discuss the implications of that fact with him urgently. He will understand."

"Yessir," concurred the Third Officer, his face lighting up with hope at the prospect, and he shot off with alacrity; out of the side door to the bridge.

When he had gone, the Captain visibly relaxed for the first time since the explosion occurred at eleven-forty; almost two hours ago. It seemed like a lifetime had passed since then, but in a few minutes, he could put the world straight, and go to his end with dignity and a clear conscience: desirous of meeting his Maker with no more guilt that he already carried for his part in the tragedy, and the responsibility for the deaths of the majority of the souls who had sailed on his ship, and who had been in his care.

The temptation of seeing Collapsible C being fitted into the davits was too much for the Chairman, and he decided it was well past time to see to his own safety. He waited for the boat to come level with the deck, and then strode towards it determinedly; glaring furiously at the Officer-in-Charge, in case the man decided to restrain him.

The restraint came, unexpectedly, from behind, in the shape of vice-like fingers which grabbed his upper arm painfully.

"What the devil...?" snapped the Chairman angrily and turned to look at his arrestor: a well built man in stoker's overalls who wore a decisive expression. The stoker had thrust his face so close, the Chairman could see the lines of his face were blackened with soot and the pores of his skin were ingrained with particles of coal-dust.

"No ye don't, yer honour," whispered his tormentor quietly: pearly white teeth flashing in the lower half of his dark visage. The Chairman struggled to free himself from the tight grip without effect.

"Take your hands off me... damn you!" he spluttered.

"No, sorr," said Declan Reilly resolutely. "If yer goin' to doi loike de rist of os, den oi'm happy to doi wit' yer. Bot if yer goin' ta save yerself, yer honour, den you'll jist have ta save me as well." Declan tapped his left temple with the index finger of his spare hand. "Oi'm de stoker from Nomber Foive, yer see, an' oi know too motch."

"Well die then, and take your knowledge with you," snarled the Chairman ungraciously; still trying to wrench himself away. The grip did not give an inch and nor did Declan; seeing himself onto a very good thing. The big Irishman shook his head and grinned inanely.

"Loife jist isn't loike dat, yer honour," he explained. "If yer go, an' oi have ta stay behind, den oi'l mek it me business to till ivryone oi can foind, exactly what did happen to de ship: just how de bunker blew oop, an' how oi saw de oiceberg miss os complete... "

"You saw the iceberg?" asked the Chairman incredulously.

"Wit' me own two oiyes, sorr: from de fo's'cle: skatin' down de soide of de ship, it was, wit' nivver a bomp or bang to worry os; de Saints preserve os, yer honour." Declan looked exceptionally pleased with his skillful disclosure.

The Chairman listened to the Irishman's words intently, and found himself hoist on his own petard! He could not take the considerable risk of leaving the stoker behind, in case he survived to give evidence, or carried out his ominous threat before the ship sank: wrecking carefully laid contingency plans, designed to limit damage to the slightest degree possible. There was no time for further argument, or any point, as Collapsible C was filling up rapidly with anxious passengers.

"Come along, my man," said the Chairman quite casually; his decision made. He started forward again, towards the lifeboat, towing Declan along behind; still attached by a hold he would not loosen until he was safely away in the boat.

The First Officer made a half-hearted attempt to bar the Chairman's way but backed down in the discharge of outrage which poured from the Chairman's mouth.

"I am the Chairman of this Line, and will be sorely needed in the aftermath of this disaster." The First Officer made to move on Declan instead. The Chairman glowered at his employee. "This man is a valuable witness and will be coming with me," he snarled in conclusion, and then swept past to claim a seat in the boat.

It was not until the collapsible touched the water that Declan let go of the Chairman's arm.

"God Bliss yer, yer honour," he muttered gratefully. It was only a temporary aberration, engendered by great relief, and the Irishman would recover his temerity soon enough. He would soon come to press for a series of rewards which would help to cloud his memories of the night's events, and keep them dulled: even creating delusions in his mind, of what he actually saw; to be offered in evidence later, at a subsequent inquiry.

At one-forty-five am, Jack Phillips would send the following message in desperation: "Engine room full up to the boilers." The *Titanic* was perilously close to her end, and those who heard could do nothing to help. The water continued to flood in and the sheer weight of it dragged her inexorably down towards her grave. The vast bubble of air, still trapped in the stern, continued to hold up that end, and the strain was severely weakening the brittle plates at the stress point of her unnatural position. The steel began to buckle and stretch along the seams, and several new cascades started up along her length. The rigid frames inside her complained and sighed under the pressure of immense forces, as if she were a wooden sailing ship, creaking and groaning, under the press of full sail. Elemental forces were merely toying with humanly constructed resistance, and, soon, something must give, as it always did in the face of nature. The Gods of the Sea could afford to laugh at man's puny efforts to conquer them!

When Benjamin Guggenheim, the ageing playboy, perceived there was no place for him in the lifeboats, he treated the whole episode as nothing more than a passing annoyance. He went back down to his stateroom and changed from the warm sweater he had donned earlier, on receiving a warning from the steward, and his life-belt, and clothed himself in evening dress: stiff collar; cravat; gold studs; the full works.

He returned to the deck to watch the last of the eligible passengers going away, and was heard to remark, to one of his fellow passengers, "If I am going to perish with this damn ship, I might as well die as I have lived: suitably attired to meet any eventuality." He was unfortunate! He had been missed by the Chairman when not pushing himself to the fore, unlike many of his fellow socialites.

Another person whose luck ran out was Colonel John Jacob Astor. He had delayed overlong in the warmth of the Gymnasium, while waiting to board the boats, and had missed the Chairman's beneficence of a reserved place. He had taken his young, pregnant bride into the gym to comfort her and cocoon her from the crush outside. At the age of forty-five, and at the top of the materialistic American social scale because of his wealth, which came chiefly from a chain of hotels, he had been involved in an acrimonious divorce over the eighteen year-old Madeleine, who he had subsequently married. They were returning from a long sojourn in Europe and Egypt, where they had been hiding from inquisitive reporters hired by several intrusive New York Editors to track them down for an exclusive story. Colonel Astor was so much in love, he did not wish for Madeleine to be exposed, even here or at this time, and as a consequence had literally missed the boat. He had tried to calm his terrified wife by explaining how she could not possibly sink, a personal phobia, as the life-jackets were filled with cork, and even went as far as to cut one open, with his pocket knife, as a demonstration of their exceptional buoyancy. When he believed she was tranquil enough to face the coming ordeal, he took her out and saw her loaded into a port-side boat by a blue-uniformed officer.

"May I join my wife?" he asked, and then continued by way of explanation, "She is so young, you see, and pregnant... I don't know how she will cope without me."

"No, Sir," replied the Second Officer adamantly. "No men are allowed in these boats until the women and children are loaded first." John Astor's eyes flared briefly: he was not used to being refused his heart's desires.

"What number is this boat?" he demanded bluntly.

"Port No. 4, sir," the Second Officer told him, believing he would lodge a complaint further up the chain of command, as such men usually do. Astor watched as the boat fell away, only two-thirds full: never taking his eyes off his wife until she disappeared from view. Then he turned to the officer and said quietly.

"I wanted to know what boat she is in... in case I survive." He turned and wandered away, disconsolately, and would come to terms with his fate like the gentleman he was.

The Third Officer returned to the bridge alone and made his report to the Captain.

"I'm sorry, sir, but the Chairman has gone."

"Gone!" roared the Captain. "What do you mean, Mister, he has gone?"

"He has gone, sir. He left in one of the collapsible boats, only a few minutes since, according to the First Officer."

"Oh, you bloody swine!" exploded the Captain, then noticed the Third Officer was looking at him curiously. He calmed down instantly. "Carry on, Third," he said and turned away to experience his anger on his own. So the damn man had bamboozled him all along, never intending to die as he had so gallantly offered. The Captain realised he should have known better, and made sure by confining the Chairman long before, whatever the consequences to himself then he should have known better about a lot of things; too late to put right now. It galled him, immensely, to think the Chairman had escaped a fate he had personally condemned so many to, and just went to show what sort of a man he was; despicable, conniving, a damn crook! There was nothing to be done about that now but at least the Captain felt he could put the record straight at last, and began to move towards the Marconi Room to send out a message containing the truth, for all the world to hear.

He had not gone more than a few yards when he perceived he was still in an untenable position. With the Chairman gone, and in a position to say anything, what was to prevent him from saying what he liked about his employee, if the Captain tried to spill the beans? That the man had cracked under the pressure and had gone mad, suffering delusions which had led him to allow the ship to collide with the iceberg in the first place - it would appear such behaviour was not beyond the Chairman. The Captain was furious, in his cleft stick, and would have kicked the timber panelling of the bridge in temper if the Third Officer had not been watching him, so he vented his frustration by clenching his fists, hidden in his greatcoat pockets, until the bones hurt, and the skin felt like it would split - he could hardly afford to let anyone see him lose control in case they survived and came to support the Chairman's stories about him. He had seldom felt so angry, or badly in his many years at sea. If he could have brought the Chairman back here, by some miracle, he would have cheerfully torn him limb from limb, despite his humanitarian beliefs. Then he had no time for further reflection; he could see how close the ship was to its end, and recognised he still had things to do: responsibilities to carry out.

He continued on, as he had started, towards the wireless room. Jack Phillips was still sending frantically, and Harold Bride stood at his shoulder, watching his every move.

"Have you raised that damned ship yet?" the Captain demanded.

"No, Sir," replied Phillips. "I am still trying."

"There no longer seems to be any point as the ship only has moments to live," murmured the Captain sorrowfully. "You are not members of my crew and have done your duty, and more, for which I thank you. It is now every man for himself and you are free to go, and may God go with you both."

Harold Bride dived into the adjoining sleeping cabin and grabbed his life-belt. He was already rushing out onto the Boat Deck when Jack Phillips told the Captain, "I think I will keep trying while the power lasts, sir, if you don't mind. It might just make the difference if I can raise that ship."

"As you wish," said the Captain as he left, knowing the Senior Operator still held himself responsible for brushing off the steamer which had tried to contact them earlier, and must still be close. It was the sort of loyalty he had always admired and could not countermand.

He made his way back to his station on the bridge.

"Third, Sixth, Quartermaster: off you go; it is every man for himself and good luck."

"But the steamer you said was close... Surely there is a chance?" protested the Third Officer.

"There is no steamer... I was mistaken," the Captain confessed with a sigh. "Now off you go, lads, and smartly now: you'll have a better chance out in the open. Jump overboard and get away from the ship while you can, before she sucks you down with her."

"Are you not coming, sir?" the Sixth Officer inquired.

"No, I think not: I am too old for swimming. Now, off you go before you miss your chance. I still have some things to do." He turned away and did not watch them go; looking out over the sinking bow, alone with thoughts of his home and family; hoping they would be spared any stain of disgrace because he had kept his bargain with a man he could not trust: praying the Chairman would spare his good name: desperately sorrowful his full life should end like this. It was not much reward for all the good things he had done in his time.

The two officers and the seaman were loath to run off and leave him, but he was already an island of preoccupation, and they recognised his right, as the Master, to go down with his ship. There was nothing more to be said.

Tom and David were eventually forced back by the rising sea. They had broken through two locked gates and proceeded as far as the First Class staterooms, directly under the bridge, only to encounter water lapping in the passageways. The deck beneath their feet angled down into deeper ponds of the greasy liquid, already strewn with floating dross: the sort of trash twentieth-century man always seems to create wherever he goes. It was obviously dangerous to go on, and they could find no way around, which was not similarly blocked. They abandoned their unfruitful search and returned topside; pausing only to snatch life-belts from one of the deserted cabins.

The last of the lifeboats was going away as they surfaced, once more, on the Boat Deck. Only Collapsible A remained, upside down on the roof of the Officers' Quarters, although efforts were being made to bring it down, for fitting into the davits. There was obviously no room for them as women still dotted the waiting crowd.

Tom was beginning to appear more and more depressed as the realisation of what he had been doing when he should have been looking to Amy, and the children's, safety, began to weigh heavily on him. David noticed his new friend's afflicted demeanour.

"Don't take on so, old chap! Look on the bright side as I have done," he counselled, and then continued, consolingly, "You will have to assume, as I have, that your wife and children have been safely loaded into one of the boats before you arrived, and are probably watching you from out there, somewhere, in a much better predicament than you find yourself forced to accept."

"Vat's alwight fir yoo, but ya ain't 'ad no effin' bars keepin' yore missus aut, 'ave ya?" complained Tom; taking his own heartfelt failings out on the system. David would not accept the censure.

"It is hardly my fault: I did not turn the keys in the locks," he objected. Tom's defiant shoulders slumped.

"Sorry, guv: it ain't ya fault." He grinned sheepishly. "I gotta big mouf, vat's all." David passed over the apology lightly.

"What do we do now, old chap?" He looked down the length of the tilting, listing liner. "I do not think she can last much longer and we seem to have run out of places to go!"

"We kin allus jamp overboard, guv," suggested Tom; back to his normal self; coming to terms with the fact that he was unable to do anything about Amy's situation if she had not made the lifeboats. David looked over the rail askance.

"Is that wise? It is rather a long way down to the sea," he commented, feeling his aching ribs tenderly.

"We 'asn't gotta lotta choice. If we stay 'ere, we're gunna end up in va water any'ow. Better we go naa, while we've gotta a chance of reachin' vem 'alf-fulled lifeboats," Tom proposed, looking around at the massed passengers ranged behind them, and adding cheekily, "before vem ouver buggers do!" Try as he might, David could not find much wrong with those sentiments.

The unlikely pair walked to the rail together.

"Per'aps we'll find va boats arr missuses is in, whiff a bitta luck... eh, guv?" Tom chattered on to keep the fear of the long drop from overcoming his optimistic intentions. David clambered up onto the rail with Tom beside him.

"Well, good luck, old chap," he offered, holding out his hand for a farewell shake.

"Gor bless ya, guv," Tom replied, locking onto the proffered grip, and holding for longer than was really necessary, "and fanks agin... Ya know wot, guv, yore alwight... fir a toff." David ignored the compliment, taking back his hand as he needed it to steady himself as he crouched on a precarious roost.

"What should us Englishmen say at a time like this?" he asked the night solemnly.

"Gawd save va King," shouted Tom foolishly, heady with sudden vertigo.

Both men jumped, simultaneously, into the dark abyss.

At two eighteen am, on the 15th April, 1912, the *Titanic* gave up the struggle to stay afloat. Her bow dipped below the surface of the ocean, and the lights, which had been kept going for so long, blinked once and went out. The bow sagged as the water clutched at her, and tautly-stretched seams began to rend. The second funnel, large enough for a train to pass through, toppled over and fell into the water, crushing several swimmers. A ghostly, tinkling sound was heard by the survivors in the boats; which was made by all the loose items, in the ship - glass, iron, china, tin, and even silver and gold, rushing forwards with the steep careen, to crash into the bulkheads, forrard. Seconds later, the complete stern section split off in a clean fracture along the stress line, and the bow, and a six hundred foot length of the hull, now freed, started a downward dive, which would last several minutes, while it plunged two-and-a-half miles to the bottom; there to embed itself in the Newfoundland Ridge.

The stern righted itself, after the schism, and bobbed about on the surface like a cork, suddenly released from the great weight of the bow, until the water flooding into it, through the gaping rift, vanquishing its skittish motions, and lashing it down with powerful bonds. Tardily, it lifted up its giant propellers, clear out of the water, and showed the name on the stern to the night sky, then started a final plunge of its own, spiralling down to come to rest, some distance from the bow, on the muddy bottom. The impact would almost destroy the stern, collapsing the layers of decks down on top of each other, while the bow would survive almost intact, by virtue of its more controlled descent. All manner of detritus would be thrown out of each part, through the cavernous holes, and came to rest on the bottom, between the two segments; creating an extensive debris field - a treasure hunter's dream! She would lie there undisturbed - while all organic material inside her was consumed by marine molluscs, and iron-eating bacteria constructed giant rusticles on her steelwork - for seventy-three years, before the ingenuity, and advancement of man, made it possible for her to be viewed again, in a state much less glamorous than the original...

The Captain was still on the bridge, unmoving, when the *Titanic* started her fatal plunge; hands in greatcoat pockets, uniform cap on head; frowning furiously, through the bridge windows, at an ocean which dared to claim his vessel. Although he had never liked her, a bond had developed during his short command, as it always does between Master and vessel, and he did not want to witness her dying like this, helpless.

He would be spared the humiliation of a lingering, or painful death by the sea, which had been his consort for so long. The millions of tons of water, which cascaded onto the bridge, as the bow went down, smashed the elegant structure to matchwood, crushing the fabric as if it were made of card, and the Captain with it. He was dead in an instant...

Lucas Meredith had just finished his book, and had put it down, to close his eyes and cogitate on the dream-world he had been in; where life was straight-forward and ordered, according to his favourite author's style. He felt the *Titanic* begin to move under his feet and thought for a moment the crew had put right whatever it was that ailed her, and that they were proceeding with the voyage. It was an idle thought. He knew, from the angle of her deck, there was only one place she would go, and it would not be her propellers that drove her there. He sat in his chair, hands clasped on the arms, facing towards the bow and prepared to enjoy the death-ride as best he could;

wagering with himself on how long it would be before the icy water engulfed him with its merciful release from the rigours of a harsh, unfriendly life, full of adversity and bad feeling. It was the last bet he would enjoy...

Thomas Andrews stood in the First Class Smoking Room, keeping himself to himself, away from the other no-hopers who had gathered there, calmly waiting for the end. He appeared, still, fascinated by the stained-glass panel depicting the sailing ship, at which he had been staring overlong. In fact, he was contemplating the ingenuousness of man in bringing the crafting of boats from hide-covered frames to the gigantic steel monstrosities, such as the one on which he stood, in a relatively short space of time within the parameters of the world's great age. Sail represented the golden age to him, when each voyage was an adventure, and all the great discoveries had been made, as opposed to this time, when ships were steam-powered barges of great size, specifically designed to move cargo, and people about, from place to place, in the shortest possible time. Sailing adventures had taken two or three years at a time, whereas today, any ship which could not cross the Atlantic in under seven days was disadvantaged in the race for paying customers or freight. It was a vicious circle really, he decided: each new invention raised the pace of life slightly, and each little step up in pace demanded new inventions to sustain it! Where it all might end was not a conclusion he was prepared to explore, and then, in the present circumstances, there was no point in viewing the future with any great excitement.

Andrews had just come around to thinking, whereas Isambard Brunel had dragged the maritime world into an era it was not quite ready for, with his steam-powered, iron ships, he himself would rather not have been part of it - regarding the designing of graceful, wooden vessels as a much more worthwhile life's work - when the deck tipped sharply beneath his feet, and the *Titanic* started her roller-coaster ride into the forbidding depths. He had little enough time left for anything, let alone profound thought...

David Peacock landed all wrong, after he had tumbled through the air from the Boat Deck, and the surface tension of the sea slammed into him when he broke through, as if he had been kicked in his already-damaged ribs by a powerful carthorse. However, the pain of it was as nothing compared to the agony of the steel bands which tightened around his torso as the icy cold did its deadly work. He sunk down deep into the water, sucking in great gulps of spume, his violent passage created, as his oxygen-starved lungs fought for the breath which had been knocked out of him on impact with the sea. The freezing saline fluid seared the delicate tissue of his lungs, as if it were scalding, and he might have gone on down, and died then, had it not been for the cork float in his life-belt, which hauled him back to the surface unceremoniously. He lay in the gentle swell, on the edge of consciousness and oblivious to everything around him - supported by his life-saving jacket.

Tom Pirbright fared a deal better. He went into the sea feet first, having had the good sense to keep his mouth tight shut; his stuffed-up nose denying the water, and the cold ingress to his vitals. He bobbed back up to the surface with his natural life-support system intact. The first thing he saw was the gentleman who had jumped with him, lying helpless in the sea, and close to death by the look of him. Tom's initial instinct was to swim away towards the lifeboats, hurriedly; giving in to his inherent predisposition for self-preservation, but he paused at David's side. The man had offered a lifeline to him once, then subsequently tried to help him, when the gentleman's understandable nature must have been urging otherwise; which demanded some sort of loyalty.

"Ya betta come alonga me, guv," he called out, and then checked his imprudence; in case he might be in need of the breath later; breath he could not afford to waste. Tom reached out and grabbed David by the scruff of the life-jacket and began to tow him away, from the sheer side of the liner, with a makeshift, one-handed dog-paddle; kicking out, feebly, with legs the overwhelming cold threatened to paralyse.

He witnessed the death throes of the *Titanic;* seeing her break up and the bow section disappear: watching, horrified, as the stern bobbed about before standing upright and then sinking into the depths: wincing with fright as the huge funnel fell into the sea not far from where he swam. When she had gone, the sea, where she had been, was littered with floating debris, and surprised passengers, unceremoniously jettisoned by the vanishing liner: the flotsam and jetsam of the tragedy! An eerie sound rose up from that dismal site; a sound fit to mortify the soul. It was anguished wailing, and the plaintive pleas for help, from the sea of abandoned human rubble;

consolidating to form a harrowing chorus of despair. It would last for some time, but would be extinguished by the sadistic cold, long before the *Carpathia,* still on her way to the scene, hove into view of the lifeboats.

Tom, burdened as he was by David, and losing his own battle with the marrow-chilling water, did not reach a safe haven until well after the *Titanic's* death. Too tired to see where he was going, he literally bumped into Port-side No 8, coxed by the Countess of Rothes. Eager female hands sought to drag him onboard, and numbed, and hardly able to move, he was well prepared to give himself up to them. Yet, once again, he delayed to see to the welfare of his helpless charge.

When he examined David closely, he realised the man was too still, too relaxed to contain any life, but still he tried to rouse his erstwhile, if short-lived, friend.

"C'mon, guv: doan' gi' up an us naa," he pleaded. "We're in vis tagivver an' sa close ta safety: get inta va boat, will ya, vere's a good man." No response greeted his words. If he could have made out David's eyes, he would have observed they were wide open; serenely set: expired. Sadly Tom pushed the corpse away, and watched the white canvas life-jacket, the only thing he could see clearly in the gloom, float off in the darkness.

"Good-bye, guv, and good luck," he murmured and gave himself up to the caring hands above, which grabbed and plucked at his life-belt.

THE AFTERMATH

The *Carpathia* rode quietly in the sea above the *Titanic's* grave. The elements were still; as if paying homage to a brave, vanquished foe. The Cunarder had come upon the lifeboats unexpectedly; some distance from the *Titanic's* broadcast position. Fortuitously, for the Chairman of the White Star Line, no one thought to fix the exact position; putting any discrepancy in the coordinates down to drift. No icebergs lingered here, but the ocean all around the *Carpathia* was littered with small chips of decaying ice, and no one would ever question the Chairman's assertion, that the *Titanic* had hit an iceberg while sailing at full speed; too ungainly and ponderous to manoeuvre her way out of danger in the time available: the evidence was manifest to all who had no reason to disbelieve the tale. The Official Board of Trade Inquiry would deem the loss accidental and recommend 'more watertight compartments in ocean-going vessels, the provision of lifeboats for all on board, and a better look-out to be kept in future' - the first two being plain common sense, but the third not easy to implement in an age before radar, sonar and asdic, and night-sight binoculars. Even the spectacle of debris, floating in the water all around, from a ship supposed to have sunk ten miles to the northwest, did not ring any warning bells in Captain Rostran's mind: he judged it to have drifted from the wreck-site with the lifeboats.

A service was being held, in the *Carpathia's* First Class Lounge, by an itinerant clergyman, travelling on the ship, who did not seem to know if it was a Requiem for the dead or Thanksgiving for those who had survived. He alternately waxed and waned, in dulcet tones, over praise for the Lord's mysterious ways and the disparaging of them; constantly reminding his bedraggled congregation it was not for mortal man to understand the workings of the Godhead's mind.

"Many are called and many are chosen," was his theme, and his unbridled joy at not being one of them was clearly evident. Three people who had lost something dear, stood together unwittingly; unrelated but not entirely unconnected.

Tom Pirbright - draped in a thick blanket to counteract the cold which had invaded his bones - had lost his wife and children. He had checked every woman among the survivors, and asked hundreds of anxious questions, but Amy was not on board, and no one could say what fate had overtaken her. He was not a religious man but had come here, to the service, in the hope of obtaining undeserved absolution for his costly lapse, and some sort of release from the guilt which would always be with him. Losing his own family was bad enough, but he had lost his brother's family too - there was no sign of Clara or her two boys either - when he had promised to protect them: the only reason Bert had left them behind; trusting them to his brother's care. Now he would have to face Bert and explain how his brother's cherished family was lost. Even if he concocted some plausible yarn, ripe with accusations of underhanded malpractice on the part of the crew, he would always have the truth on his conscience, and would have to live with it. It would only be a small part of his penance. What he would have to live with, over Amy's, and the children's loss, was a cross he did not want to bear but would be saddled with; a cross made heavier by the lead weights his costly dalliance pressed upon it. Earlier, during the service, some obscure force had made him look behind himself, and had seen Sian - her bright, titian hair tousled by seawater, a few ranks behind his frontal position. She was alone, without her alcoholic parent, and Tom could only conclude Mick had not survived. Sian was looking directly at him, as if she was the one who had summoned his attention by supernatural means. Their eyes met briefly, and she smiled at him invitingly. Tom swivelled his head desperately, to escape her gaze, and fixed his eyes on the clergyman; seeking the protection of righteousness. He shivered uncontrollably, but it was not the cold in his bones which triggered the reaction: it was revulsion. He was confused about the whole business and did not know which way to hang. He was still in shock over the loss of Amy and the children. It had not struck home yet, and he had not stumbled into the great crater which had developed as the bottom fell out of his world; it was waiting, sinisterly menacing, until the moment he allowed himself to relax.

Molly Peacock stood with her two children gathered into her skirts, and they clung to her gratefully; badly shocked by the loss of their father. She too had searched the ship, and the survivors, for her husband, without success. She would never know how David had died, even though the man who had been with him at the end stood beside her. Tom had never known David's name, and neither Molly, nor he, would ever make the connection. She too, had not yet been afflicted by the great pain which would come in time. While there was hope, she would not accept he was dead, and those close to her, and those who had lost no-one offered her this olive-branch to appease their own guilty sensations. Although all the lifeboats had been accounted for and were hanging in the *Carpathia's* davits even now, news was rife, among the survivors, that a great armada of ships was on its way to the disaster area - the *Californian* had already turned up this morning, after resuming normal wireless communications and being alerted to the tragedy, and was scouring the locality for survivors or bodies. Hypothermia was not a condition known to medical science, at the time, and while there was a chance some of the swimmers were still alive, there was definitely hope. Molly accepted all this with stoical forbearance, as was expected by her breeding, and the floods of tears, and the sense of deep loss, would not come until later, when all hope was gone. She would return to England and the comfort of her two families, David's and her own, who were used to the trauma of offering up the lives of their sons in the development of the Empire and lucrative trade. She and her children would be cossetted, and would want for nothing.

Lorna Wainwright had also lost something, although her family was intact; her self respect. When she looked around and perceived how few men had survived the catastrophe, and most of them influential, she felt very badly that she had not been called upon to make the same sacrifice as her friend, Molly; who stood beside her. It was not that she wished poor Jonathan dead; just that while she had no pain to suffer, she could not unite with those around her in mourning, and felt terribly isolated: it was a curious reaction.

She had been a tower of strength since she came aboard the *Carpathia*, being a comfort to Molly, and the chief contributor to that misguided woman's pool of faith by assuring her David was likely aboard the *Californian* right now and perfectly alright. Jonathan was not at the service. He was down below in the sick-bay, still a victim of the cataleptic state which had claimed him. He lay in a bed, deathly still and stared up at the bulkhead above him; in a secret, comfortable place where humanity could not reach him. The over-worked Ship's Doctor had little enough time to spare for Lorna, but he had given her his opinion briefly. Jonathan, he said, was in a state of deep shock, unable to accept the trauma of what had happened;

blocking it out by disconnecting his brain from the senses he possessed. He could not see, feel or hear, and did not want to until he could feel safe again. Whether the condition would respond to treatment or if it was permanent, the doctor could not say, as he was not a specialist in the field, but he knew of many cases where such patients had fully recovered after some time; with careful handling and the right kind of nursing. Perhaps, he suggested, one of the disciples of a Viennese Neurologist called Freud, who abounded in America, might be able to reach him and unlock the door to his mind. This was what had caused Lorna's distress, that her husband had been saved, because of his cabbage-like condition, when many others, better qualified, had perished. It disturbed her sense of fair play and detracted from her feeling of being one with all the other women; a sister of their terrible grief. This perverse feeling would not persist and was, in part, the manifestation of her own shock at the realisation her premonition had been right all along. In time she would come to realise how much she appreciated her husband, and loved him, and was glad he had survived, for when he recovered from his breakdown, he would emerge a much better man, outgoing and concerned for humanity, no longer a studious island; transformed like a butterfly in its chrysalis stage.

The Chairman was probably the best humoured of all the *Titanic's* survivors on that morning after the disaster; not happy, but cheered by the knowledge his deceitful master-plan had come through unscathed: the reputation of the White Star Line, and its continuance, looked assured. He was aware all publicity is good publicity, however bad it appeared to be at the time, but would never appreciate what sort of niche the *Titanic* would carve herself in history or for how long her memory would be sustained, as the first great holocaust of the twentieth century; forerunning many, much worse, which would make it the most memorable century since the emergence of man from the Stone-age.

He had sent the following message to the Company's New York office, first thing, as soon as Collapsible C had been winched inboard, and the necessary formalities, and explanations, concluded with Captain Rostron, of the *Carpathia:*

"Deeply regret to advise you, *Titanic* sank this morning after collision with iceberg, resulting in serious loss of life. Full particulars to follow later."

He had gone straight from the Wireless Room to find the Irishman, from last night, who knew too much for his own good. He found Declan Reilly eventually and set about negotiations which were very important to him, and the White Star Line. Declan was more astute than he looked, and drove a hard bargain. He settled, after some unnecessary haggling - but then he had never been in this position before and was enjoying his moment of glory over a hated English oppressor - for the price of a smallholding in Ireland; a lump sum to furnish his house and equip his land; a life pension to ensure against any future downturns - he actually said, "Jost in case dere's anudder petata famine, yer honour!" sarcastically - and First Class passage on the next Company ship going east, so he could start his new life at once. For this bounty he would sell his soul and say anything the Chairman wished him to, at any subsequent investigation or inquiry - it made no difference to him what any Englishman wished to suppress as long as he had been recompensed, personally, for what he considered to be many, many years of British misrule and injustice. The price in cash, to the Chairman, was not heavy, but the payment in pride was exorbitant, but he had no time to worry about it just then: he had a great number of instructions to pass onto Declan Reilly, and very little time on his hands.

When he had finished procuring the Irishman, the Chairman still had an urgent task to undertake. He had checked the names of the surviving crew compiled by one of Rostran's officers - avidly, and had found there was only one other person aboard who knew about the fire in Forward Coal Bunker No 5, as far as he knew, and if his original instructions had been carried out. What that man knew, and where he had been at the time of the explosion, was something the Chairman needed to find out, both urgently and desperately.

He found the Second Officer on the *Carpathia's* Promenade Deck, by the rail, looking out over the littered ocean. The officer had obviously borrowed some clothes, while his own were being dried, as the uniform he wore was too big for him, and made him look untidy. He did not hear the Chairman approach and continued to gaze into the distance, not turning his head until the Chairman spoke to him.

"Good to see you survived. Terrible... terrible disaster!" When the Second Officer faced him, the Chairman could see how pinched and drawn his features were, blue-tinged, with surprised, bloodshot eyes sunken deeply into his skull. He had obviously been in the water for some time after the *Titanic* sank.

"Yes, and such a terrible waste of life," the officer sighed, as if he were completely fatigued by life. "Only seven hundred survivors, out of triple that, is not a very good result."

"Quite... quite," agreed the Chairman, hastening on, as this was not the time or place to have such a debate. "I came to thank you for your efforts last night... on behalf of myself and the Company. I was most impressed with the way you handled the port-side lifeboats and got the passengers away." In actuality, he was not impressed at all - this officer had frustrated his plans several times during the sinking, and maintained a position he could have done without. However, until the Chairman could glean what this man knew, and how strongly he felt about it, there would be no word of censure or recrimination: that would be reserved for the future, when, with a bit of luck, he owned the man's soul.

"I was merely doing my duty, sir, and following my Skipper's orders," the Second Officer stated pompously.

"Quite... quite." Now it was time to make his play. "So many good officers were lost in this tragedy," bemoaned the Chairman, and then darted in, trying to open up his man. "I hope you are not thinking of leaving the Line or have been put off seafaring by... "

"Who me? Good Lord, no, sir. The sea is my life: I could not imagine what else I should do," protested the Second Officer, and the Chairman knew he had the man; career officers only want one thing: to end up with a ship of their own; aspiring to Godlike status, which is what a Captain is close to, when at sea.

"Ahem... mmmm." The Chairman cleared his throat. "I have taken note of your name, and as soon as I return to London I shall pass it onto our Selection Board. The Line needs competent officers, like yourself, and with my personal recommendation as to your exemplary conduct under difficult and trying circumstances, I have no doubt your career will blossom quite quickly; in a way you would not normally envisage. I would expect to see you as Master of your own ship within... shall we say a year? Do I make myself clear?"

"Yes, sir, thank you, sir. I would appreciate your patronage," bubbled the Second Officer, aware, suddenly, he was in the presence of influence and authority. It was both welcome and unexpected good news, and he wondered ironically on the old adage concerning one man's meat being another's poison: there was an analogy here somewhere, in all of this: he would gain what many of his brother officers, from the *Titanic*, had lost; a golden future.

The Chairman was emboldened by the Second Officer's somewhat craven attitude.

"Now, I need to know what you were doing when the ship struck the iceberg? Where were you, and what did you see?" he asked.

"Nothing much, I'm afraid, sir. You see, I had already retired to my bunk after my watch ended at ten. I slept through the whole thing."

"And what did the Captain say to you, when you arrived on the bridge?" The officer thought for a few moments.

"As I recall, sir, only that the ship was sinking and we, the officers, should go to boat stations, to get the women and children away."

"And how did you find out the ship had collided with an iceberg?" the Chairman wanted to know. The Second Officer considered, again, for about a half a minute.

"I cannot really say, sir: it's all a bit of a blur, really. I had just woken from a deep sleep... everyone was talking about it... I... Why, is there a problem, sir?"

"No... no... of course not," demurred the Chairman, and hurried on. "There will be an Official Board of Trade Inquiry, naturally. You, as the senior surviving officer, will bear the brunt of the questioning, as to how the disaster occurred, and will doubtless be asked to give your opinion about a great number of matters. You will have to be very clear in what you say, to anyone, and the point of these questions is to ascertain just how much you do know. I am, of course, party to all the facts. I had a full report from our late, gallant Captain, and Andrews, the designer, who inspected the damage. I shall be able to fill you in on any detail you may lack for the report you will be expected to make. The tragedy has happened, and cannot be reversed by words, ideas or inquiries. As one of the Line's future, senior officers, I am sure you can see the need to put up a united front in the face of what is to come!"

"Yes, sir," agreed the Second Officer, fully aware.

"There is one more thing," continued the Chairman, "the fire in that coal bunker..."

"Surely it was put out?" offered the Second Officer.

"Quite so... quite so, but I do not see the need to mention it at all, do you? I see no point in exposing ourselves to rumour and innuendo - the press is always quick to fasten onto that - and idle speculation has a way of doing some sort of harm, in the long run. Do you understand me?"

"Absolutely," commented the Second Officer.

"Good... good," uttered the Chairman and relaxed visibly. "I think we understand each other! We will speak again... soon... before we arrive in New York. Now, you must excuse me: I have other pressing matters to attend." The Chairman turned, without another word, and walked away. The press would vilify him for saving himself at the expense of others - giving him the epithet 'Brute'; which was a lampoon of his name; while the Captain would be glorified for going down with the ship, in the tradition of the sea - and what he had done in the last twelve hours would sour the sweet taste of success he had enjoyed for so long.

After he had gone, the Second Officer turned away from the rail with a bad taste in his mouth. He had accepted the Chairman's offer, but did not like himself for it very much, and he did not feel particularly good about things. He recalled last Saturday night, on the bridge, when he heard about Lucas Meredith and his cheating, and remembered clearly just what he had thought about the man. He grimaced as he realised he, himself, had become that thing which he overly despised - a rogue and a cheat!

THE END

POSTSCRIPT

Article from the Classic Ships Monthly in September 1993

The Titanic:- Tragic accident or massive fraud?

I saw a television programme the other night, 'The Treasures of the Titanic', which raised a lot of questions in my mind although this was not the intention of the film. Has the first and last voyage of this noble ship become the stuff of legend: a myth created by the media to unwittingly justify a nefarious incident which has never leaked out? Does someone, anyone, hide a dusty file containing guilty secrets about an avoidable disaster?

Let us consider the facts as they are generally known. The *Titanic*, declared to be unsinkable by its makers, owners and the press, by virtue of its watertight compartments, sank on its maiden voyage, after a collision with an iceberg, three hundred miles off the coast of Newfoundland, on 14-15th April 1912, with the loss of 1,522 lives. Everyone knows not enough lifeboats had been provided to take off the passengers and crew, and many heroic sacrifices were made by those who remained on board, to see the women and children safely away in the boats, while the ship's orchestra played manfully on, to maintain an atmosphere of calm, in true British and American style, full of grit and stiff upper-lip. An act of God, you might say, or was it? Could the whole scenario, the sacrifice, the loss of life, have been averted?

An American gentleman on the programme I saw, related how his father had served in the Great War, with a man who had sailed on a merchant ship, after the tragedy, with a stoker who had survived the disaster. The stoker claimed a fire had been burning in one of the liner's coal bunkers since she sailed from Queenstown in Northern Ireland. Why was this fire allowed to burn? Presumably, because it would have created a long delay while the bunker, containing thousands of tons of coal, was cleaned out; the fire dealt with; and then refilled: not an auspicious start to the cruising career of a supership, the largest man-made artefact on the face of the earth at the time. It was not an admission the vain owners would have wanted to make regarding the *Titanic*, the epitome of reliability and sumptuousness, as they claimed. Such a revelation would hardly endorse dependability or invulnerability; criteria they sought to encourage in the hope of procuring bookings at the expense of their rivals. How was the fire contained? More than likely it was kept damped down with a water spray - the stoker never said and no other surviving crew member has admitted knowledge of the incendiary coal - until such time as the fuel was consumed, in the furnaces, and the seat of the smouldering fire reached; to be dealt with without inconvenience to the rich, First Class passengers, or the owner's vanity. Maybe it was not common knowledge, and the bunker remained battened down to starve the fire of oxygen in an attempt to make it burn itself out. Smouldering coal produces a highly flammable gas, used in domestic appliances before the discovery of organic methane under the North Sea: any spark could have set off a devastating explosion!

After the wreck of the *Titanic* was located by Dr Robert Ballard, the hull was examined, by a subsequent Franco-American expedition, on the submersible Nautile at a depth of 12,500 feet where it lies under the ocean. The mini-submarine found, not a long gash running down the length of the hull as might be expected in a collision with an iceberg, but a round hole, thirty feet across, consistent with an internal explosion blowing out the hull plates, roughly corresponding to the site of one of the coal bunkers, or so the programme indicated. No one present in the sub was sufficiently qualified to confirm this was the case and, of course, considering the pressures involved at that sort of depth, no expert will ever be able to examine the large puncture in the ship's side at close range. Could the iceberg have inflicted such a puncture? Not in the way the collision was described by the surviving crewmen.

That the *Titanic* had a brush with an iceberg is not disputed; it is the seriousness of this brush which is. At 11.40 pm on 14th April, the lookouts, Fred Fleet and Reginald Lee, spotted an iceberg 500 yards ahead - it apparently appeared suddenly at this range on a clear night. They immediately rang the warning bell in the crows-nest and telephoned the bridge. The First Officer, Mr Murdock, ordered the helmsman to put the wheel 'hard-a-starboard'. The *Titanic*, sailing along at twenty knots, veered to port. Mr Murdock ordered the engines stopped, and then put into reverse. In the event, a head-on strike was avoided and the iceberg brushed along the starboard side of the ship, or so it was stated. At twenty knots, the reported speed, the ship would have covered the distance in around forty-five seconds; hardly time for evasive action to have been taken; the huge engines stopped and put into reverse; remembering the ship was three hundred yards long. The impact was not noticed by many of the passengers, and none were on deck; it was a bitterly cold night. Only the crew were aware of the collision. Laurence Beesley, a surviving passenger said, "There came, what seemed to me, nothing more than an extra heave of the engines, and the more than usual, obvious dancing motion of the mattress on which I sat. Nothing more than that - no sound of a crash or anything else; no sense of shock, no jar that felt like one heavy body meeting another." After this Beesley, a young science teacher, returned to his reading. Does this description convey the impression of an immovable iceberg scraping its way down the 882ft length of an unsinkable liner, gouging it open like a tin can, or is it more consistent with an explosion, of trapped gas in a confined space, popping out the rivets in the plates of a mortal ship to create a hole; and the resulting inrush of water? Dr Ballard found no evidence of a large gash in the *Titanic's* side, only a few buckled, punctured plates which he maintains, in his book, is 'possible ice damage; creased plates with horizontally opened seams.' Any other damage, he says, is conveniently buried under sixty feet of mud into which the bow embedded itself on its fatal dive to the bottom. However, these buckled plates occur just abaft the point where the bows bent away from the bulk of the hull on impact with the seabed and could be no more than stress fractures; not iceberg damage at all. No other damage is evident in any of the photographs taken, apart from the large hole reported by the crew of the *Nautile*. The unfortunate ship took only two hours to sink.

Edward Wilding, a naval architect from the *Titanic's* makers, Harland and Wolff, calculated the amount of water required to sink the ship, in the time it took, for the Official Inquiry. Using a formula to arrive at the size of the hole needed to flood the ship to that lethal extent, despite its watertight compartments, he came up with a figure of 12 sq ft; much less than the 30ft hole photographed by the *Nautile*. The English naval architect, K C Barnaby, contends in his book,

'Some Ship Disasters and Their Causes', that the fatal damage to the two ships, the *Andrea Doria* in 1956, and the *Shillong* in 1957, would have been no more than a nuisance to the *Titanic*. The fault lay not in the soundness of the *Titanic's* construction, but in her inability to withstand the hammer blow to her vitals which an explosion below the waterline, like a torpedo strike from the inflammable coal gas, might have given her. (It is not widely reported a sister-ship, the *Britannia*, was sunk by a German mine - a single explosion! - during the Great War while serving as a hospital ship; this vessel, a faithful copy of the *Titanic's* design, also had watertight compartments. In 1992, Dr Ballard found the wreck of the *Lusitania* off the coast of Ireland, in relatively shallow water. He put the reason for her sinking down to a massive explosion in a starboard coal bunker, caused by a German torpedo igniting volatile coal dust when it struck the ship. She too had watertight compartments and sank in twenty minutes!)

Then there is the case of the unfortunate Captain Stanley Lord, Master of the *Californian*, vilified during his lifetime, and after his death - I understand his son still seeks to clear his name to this day - for not coming to the aid of the stricken *Titanic* while she sank. The *Californian* was reputed to be between ten and nineteen miles north-northeast of the *Titanic's* last reported position - the only ship, possibly, in visual contact. He was accused of failing to recognise the distress rockets of the sinking liner for what they were, and for refusing to take action which could have saved many lives. Captain Lord asserted, until his dying day, the ship he saw firing rockets was not a passenger ship at all - he had already warned the *Titanic* of icebergs ahead, having been rebuffed by the over-worked radio operator, and had stopped his own ship for the night, not expecting the *Titanic* to charge on towards the ice-flows at a speed of twenty knots. Was he ever near enough to see the *Titanic* from his position?

Dr Ballard, during his quest in 1985, started his search at the liner's last known position and, after covering the whole area in a box-grid pattern, eventually found the wreck 10-12 nautical miles, approx, southeast of her last reported location - for the supporters of Captain Lord, this could have put the *Californian* anything up to 25 - 30 miles away, depending on drift, and surely out of visual range. The explanation for this discrepancy is given as: the *Titanic's* officers calculated her speed at twenty-two knots when she was only doing twenty; putting her projected position further west than imagined - is this likely on the most modern ship of her day? Other explanations include drift - ten nautical miles in two hours? (The lifeboats from the stricken liner were found by the *Carpathia* only five miles southwest, from the actual site of the wreck, four hours later - an indication of the true rate of drift.) The *Titanic's* engine telegraph was found, by the *Nautile*, - via a remote-controlled camera module which managed to penetrate the hull of the ship through the fracture, where she had broken in half - to be at slow ahead while the bridge telegraph showed full stop - the reason being given that no one was left in the engine-room to shut off the engines in answer to the last frantic order. To cover ten miles in two hours, the liner must have turned around and steamed at the rate of five knots while rapidly filling with water, or to have gone backwards, which is not born out by the engine-room telegraph - hardly possible in the arduous circumstances!

Now we come to the lifeboats themselves. The original designer of the ship, Alexander Carlisle, had suggested sixty-four boats would be required for such a gigantic vessel. For reasons of vanity, or economy (this hardly seems likely as the ship was lavishly decorated and equipped almost to the point of absurdity) only sixteen lifeboats were finally installed, plus four collapsible lifeboats, on the reputedly unsinkable ship, conforming to outdated British Board of Trade regulations; or was it something else, like a direct challenge to the elements by a Boardroom of Directors who should have known better - surely the final responsibility for this imperceptive decision rested with them? Calculations reveal that only 705 out of 2227 passengers and crew survived the disaster and sixty lifeboats would have been, pro-rata, the correct number to carry. Was Alexander Carlisle that far out in his original calculations?

What are we left with? An unsinkable liner with a dangerous fire in its belly, apparently in collision with an iceberg, that none of the passengers saw, sank 10-12 miles southeast of her last reported position - all very convenient for the owners in an insurance claim, against Lloyds of London, for millions of pounds at today's values! Now all the principal actors in the drama are dead and the White Star Line gone, I can ask the questions which trouble me. Was this tragedy an accident or the sort of gross negligence Captain Lord, of the *Californian* has always had laid at his door, perpetrated by certain guilty people in a conspiracy of silence? Did Captain Smith, the Master of the *Titanic*, know there was a smouldering fire aboard his ship? Did he make any representations to his owners about putting it out, possibly delaying the maiden voyage for a couple of days, and admitting susceptibility to error? The voyage had already been put back once after her sister-ship, the *Olympic*, had been involved in a collision. Was the stoker telling the truth? Was a fire really smouldering in a coal bunker? Did an iceberg strike the ship a mortal blow? Why did none of the surviving passengers see it? They could not all have been in bed. Was there an iceberg at all? Did the crew lie to protect their futures with the Company? Why was a false position reported by the Radio Officer in his distress calls? Was he given an inaccurate position, by Captain Smith, in a loyal attempt to protect the owners; to avoid the ship ever being found, and the truth coming out? It seems to me, an iceberg striking a ship is an accident: a clandestine fire in a ship with insufficient lifeboats to carry away all those on board is an act of gross negligence, likely to have put the White Star Line out of business if claims for millions of pounds in compensation from those who survived, and the families of those who perished, had ever been brought into civil court. Was this a massive fraud effected by greedy owners, with the connivance of the Captain and crew, to avoid payment of compensation, and to validate an insurance claim which might never have been met if the true facts had come out at the time? Incredibly, only three passengers were called to give evidence at the Board of Trade Inquiry during 2nd May - 3rd July 1912; Sir Cosmo and Lady Duff Gordan, and J Bruce Ismay, Chairman of the White Star Line, who had taken a place in a lifeboat for himself, and was heavily censured for his spineless action! The others giving evidence were experts, members of the crew and the ship's officers. Was poor Captain Smith, who gave up his life, got at during those last, fateful hours? Iceberg or explosion? Surely this was the most preventable of disasters! Have others, like Captain Lord, had the finger of blame pointed at them to keep its accusing castigation away from the real culprits?

The mystery is likely to remain forever, unless the *Titanic* is raised from her watery grave, 12,500 feet down in complete darkness - an unlikely event. I must leave her epitaph to a survivor, interviewed on 'that programme' which started all of this. Her mother, on finding out she would travel on the *Titanic*, confessed to having a premonition of disaster about the voyage. Her husband, assuring her of her error, reminded her of the liner's reported invincibility, of its invulnerability in the sight of God. The woman's mother replied, "Don't you think that might be pushing God a little too far?" Who is to say she was not right?

POSTSCRIPT

On 24th April 1912, the *Olympic*, *Titanic's* sister-ship was due to leave Southampton. Her 'black gang' (the stokers) went on strike. They said they would not work on a ship which did not carry enough lifeboats. Why the stokers? Why not the stewards or the seamen? Had a stoker recently arrived back in England? Did the stokers know more than anyone else? Eventually 285 crew deserted the ship and the voyage was cancelled!